THE PLANT PROGRAMME

by Professor Jane Plant CBE
and Gill Tidey

D0101333

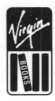

This edition first published in 2004 by
Virgin Books Ltd
Thames Wharf Studios
Rainville Road
London W6 9HA

First published in hardback in Great Britain in 2001 by
Virgin Publishing Ltd

First paperback publication by Virgin Books Ltd in 2002

A catalogue record for this book is available
from the British Library.

ISBN 978 0 7535 0952 4

Typeset by Roger Kohn Designs
Printed in the UK by CPI Bookmarque, Croydon, CR0 4TD

Contents

Acknowledgements

Both Jane and Gill want to thank their
husbands, Peter Simpson and David Falvey,
for their support and encouragement, and for
acting as part-time experimental cooks and
tasters. We would also like to thank the many
people who, knowing of the goals of the book,
offered appropriate recipes of their own.
Where these could be accommodated,
they are acknowledged with the recipe.

'Think non dairy – live non dairy'

1 Introduction

1.1 WELCOME

This book was written in response to a flood of requests for further help in implementing the Plant Programme diet. The diet, which was described in my book *Your Life in Your Hands* and subsequently in *Prostate Cancer: Understand, Prevent and Overcome*, has transformed the approach to the prevention and treatment of breast and prostate cancer. Since these books were published even more evidence has emerged on the problems caused by hormones and growth factors in milk. Some studies indicate that consuming dairy products increases the risk, not only of breast and prostate cancer, but also testicular cancer and lung cancer in men.

One of the main challenges to the diet has been the assertion that people will become calcium deficient if they do not eat dairy produce and that this will lead to osteoporosis. This is not the case. Americans and Scandinavians consume the highest amounts of dairy produce in the world, but have the highest bone fracture rates, whereas people in Asian countries consume very little dairy produce and have very low bone fracture rates. The average calcium intake is less than 300 milligrams a day in Singapore, yet the bone fracture rate there is one fifth that of the US (http://www.lightparty.com/Health/Milk.html). The Plant Programme diet will supply you with calcium from the same source that cows and hippopotami obtain theirs – from vegetable matter.

In preparing this book I have joined forces with my friend Gill Tidey to describe how everyone can make the necessary changes and adopt the 'Plant Programme' in their daily lives. My original books were about 'why', this book is about 'how' and it includes practical, comprehensive advice for healthy living and eating. It is aimed particularly at those who want to treat or prevent breast or prostate cancer and I have heard from many sufferers from these diseases telling me how much *Your Life in Your Hands* and *Prostate Cancer* has helped them. Many others have written telling me how much the advice has helped treat other illnesses including allergic conditions such as asthma and eczema and other skin problems such as psoriasis, and some auto-immune diseases and Crohn's disease. The Plant Programme is also heart healthy. Therefore, everyone can benefit from following it.

As earth scientists Gill and I have both worked and lived in many countries, particularly in Asia, where breast and prostate cancer rates are exceptionally low. We both know it is easy to create good and exciting meals that minimise the risks inherent in modern diets rich in dairy and convenience food. The ready availability of Asian ingredients now makes it easy for everyone to adopt this delicious healthy way of eating based on an 'East meets West' style, which Gill, in particular, came to love and master while cooking for her family when she lived in Australia.

Gill and I both have very busy lives: I work as Chief Scientist at the British Geological Survey and Professor of Geochemistry at Imperial College, London and Gill is the Director of the Nottingham Energy Partnership. As well as managing high level careers, we enjoy looking after our families and homes and entertaining, so we are well aware of the complexities and stresses of modern day life. We have therefore developed a cookbook based on the following principles:

- The food is healthy and nutritious
- The recipes are simple and easy to follow
- The whole way of cooking is practical and the recipes are mostly inexpensive and quick to make
- The dishes are tempting and delicious.

Within a few weeks of following the Plant Programme Diet you will probably look and feel much better and wonder how your body managed to cope with your old unhealthy ways.

Remember there is nothing strange about the diet and *do not allow yourself to be persuaded that you need dairy*. The good things in dairy produce, whether calcium or conjugated linoleic acid (CLA), come from the vegetable matter the cows eat. It is much healthier to eat vegetables yourself. Millions of people have thrived on a dairy-free diet for centuries without developing the diseases that plague rich Western societies today. Also, remember that the diet is not meant to replace conventional medical treatment for breast or prostate cancer, but to complement it in the same way that diabetics or patients with heart disease are given dietary guidance to complement their orthodox medical treatment. Indeed one of the main benefits of the diet is that it helps people to complete their treatment including chemotherapy and to take back control of their lives.

I hope that this book will help all the many people who have written to me following publication of *Your Life in Your Hands* and *Prostate Cancer* to keep to the Plant Programme and to enjoy doing so.

Jane Plant

1.2 HOW TO USE THE BOOK

Before you begin it might help if we give you a few tips on how to use the book. The first chapters give a brief outline of the rationale behind the cookbook and describe how to apply the principles of healthy eating in your life. (Although, if you want to understand fully the scientific principles behind this approach to diet, we suggest you read *Your Life in Your Hands* or *Prostate Cancer*.)

There are then chapters giving sound advice on equipping your kitchen and buying, storing and preparing healthy food. These are followed by three sections of delicious recipes for breakfasts, light meals and snacks, and main meals. All the recipes serve four people unless otherwise stated, with the exception of juice recipes, which are designed for one to two people. There are weekly meal plans both for cancer patients and those wishing to cut their risk of contracting breast or prostate cancer. There is even a section on healthy meals for kids and teenagers and a section on eating out and travelling.

Finally, there is a chapter entitled 'Food as Medicine'. This includes helpful advice on coping with the side effects of cancer treatment and other problems with health that can affect cancer sufferers and others. All the methods were 'road tested' by Jane during her illness and many of the people that she has since helped have found them useful. As in the case of the Plant Programme, the advice cannot cause harm if you use the information sensibly in combination with conventional medicine.

Those wishing to cut their risk of suffering from breast or prostate cancer can simply select the recipes they find most tempting and follow the advice on shopping and preparing food in the early sections of the book. Cancer patients should read these sections carefully and follow the scoring systems, which are there to guide them.

MEASUREMENTS

T	tablespoon
Tsp	teaspoon
L	litre
ml	millilitre
kg	kilogram
gm	gram
cm	centimetre
cup	250 ml

2 'Plant Programme' Essentials

MAKING THE CHANGES

2.1 PRINCIPLES OF THE DIET

Your Life in Your Hands explained the scientific basis of a healthy diet aimed especially at preventing and treating breast and prostate cancer. This was based on intensive research into the medical and scientific literature and statistical data on the diseases following Jane's five-times personal battle with breast cancer. if you read the first book, you will remember that Jane's cancer had spread to lymph nodes in her neck, despite a radical mastectomy, three further operations, 35 radiotherapy treatments, irradiation of her ovaries to induce the menopause and a number of chemotherapy treatments. Despite all of this she had been given only three months to live by her doctors. Jane then recalled that people in rural China, where she had worked, had a very low incidence of breast (or prostate) cancer. At that point she changed her diet and to everyone's amazement, including her own, the large cancerous lump in her neck disappeared within five weeks. By the time this book is published that will have been eight years ago.

Following that illness Jane had helped 63 other women, all of who remained cancer free. She was then persuaded to put everything she knows about the two killer diseases into a book to make the knowledge available to everyone. That book was *Your Life in Your Hands*. She subsequently followed it with *Prostate Cancer: Understand, Prevent and Overcome* and we hope you will all have read the sound scientific evidence for changing to a healthy diet in one or both of these books. We are not going to repeat the scientific basis of the diet here, but it is worth looking in a little more detail at the Eastern diet in order to understand the principles of this book.

COMPARISON OF US AND CHINESE DIETS

In some parts of China less than 3% of the population under 65 years of age die from any form of cancer, and breast and prostate cancer are almost unknown. Stomach cancer is more prevalent in China, but it is attributed by most experts to unhygienic methods of storing and preserving food. The prevalence of the disease is declining as more people use refrigerators. Typically, people in China do not eat dairy produce and the composition of their diet is very different to a typical Western diet in several other respects – for example:

● *The Chinese take in more calories than Americans do* (but are much less obese)*
● *Only 14% of calories in the average Chinese diet is from fat, compared to almost 36% in the West*
● *Animal protein makes up 11% of the diet of the average American but only 1% of the average Chinese (and a high proportion of that is from fish, eggs, chicken, duck or pork, rather than beef)*
● *Vegetables such as soya are the main source of protein in China giving a fibre intake of 34 grams a day on average with no evidence of iron or other mineral deficiency, while in the US the average fibre intake is only 10–12 grams a day*

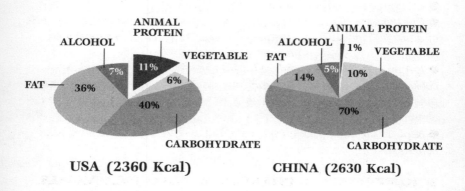

USA (2360 Kcal)   CHINA (2630 Kcal)

*From T Colin Campbell and Chen Junshi's papers on Diet and Chronic degenerative disease, published in 1994

Furthermore, in Japan a healthy diet is believed to be based on eating at least thirty different ingredients a day. Compare this with the diet of the average American, for whom 40% is from dairy.

There are several reasons why the Eastern diet is likely to prevent hormone-related cancers, but principal amongst those is that, traditionally, it contains no dairy. Milk contains growth factors and hormones known to promote breast and prostate and other types of cancer. Moreover, since the 1940s milking has been maintained even when cows are pregnant further increasing the amount of oestrogen in milk. Milk also concentrates hormone-mimicking pollutants from the environment.

The Chinese diet is also:
- *low in fat, which causes oestrogen to be released in women's bodies*
- *high in fibre, which helps to eliminate excess oestrogen from the body*
- *high in phytoestrogens which are protective against breast cancer*

The basis of the Plant Programme is:

1. TO REDUCE THE INTAKE OF NATURAL HORMONES AND GROWTH FACTORS FROM FOOD.

How?
- *Eliminate **all** dairy produce*
- *Cut down on the amount of meat eaten – it should comprise only 10% of daily intake for the prevention of cancer and should be eliminated completely by those with active cancer*
- *Eat only organically produced meat or game that is thoroughly cooked, in order to break down hormones, growth factors and pollutants (but do not burn it because this will form other damaging carcinogenic chemicals)*
- *Replace animal protein, especially dairy, with soya-based food, and cereals and pulses*

2. TO REDUCE THE INTAKE OF MAN-MADE CHEMICALS FOR WHICH THERE IS EVIDENCE FOR, OR A SUSPICION OF, CARCINOGENICITY, ESPECIALLY ENDOCRINE-DISRUPTING CHEMICALS.

These are suspected of causing cancers of the reproductive organs, including the breast and prostate, and also testicular cancer and cancer of the womb and ovaries. Endocrine-disrupting chemicals are persistent and bio-accumulate, becoming particularly concentrated in certain foods.

How?

● Avoid all dairy produce, fish liver oils and farmed fish, especially carnivorous fish such as salmon
● Eat only organically produced food, especially in the case of fat meats such as pork and duck, and even then remove the fat and the skin
● Do not use plastic, especially soft plastic wrappings, or eat food from cans with plastic linings
● Filter tap water through charcoal, then boil it and store it in glass bottles
● Drink liquids stored in glass with cork or aluminium seals, but not in plastic bottles
● Never have 'diet' drinks, or other food or drink that contains man-made sweeteners such as saccharine or aspartame

3. INCREASE THE PROPORTION OF FOOD THAT IS PROTECTIVE AGAINST CANCER

How?

● Eat as much fresh organic vegetables and fruit as possible, especially red vegetables such as tomatoes, red peppers and chillies; cruciferous vegetables such as bok choy, cauliflower and broccoli; and orange vegetables, including peppers, carrots and pumpkin
● Eat lots of fresh herbs
● Eat vegetables as fresh and raw as possible and have at least five large portions of fruit and vegetables as salads or juices every day. The UK Government recommendation of five portions a day, which includes prepared fruit and vegetables, is completely inadequate for healthy living – one portion should be at least one piece of fruit or $1/2$ cup of raw vegetables
● Eat a diet rich in phytoestrogens, including soya and other beans and peas, whole grain cereals especially flax, nuts and berries especially cranberries, and sprouting seeds especially alfalfa
● Eat spices, many of which have antioxidant properties. Turmeric, in particular, causes cancer cells to commit suicide

● *Eat lots of garlic, which has anti-cancer and other health benefits, and onions and chives*
● *Drink lots of green tea*

4. ENSURE THAT YOU CONSUME ADEQUATE QUANTITIES OF THE KEY NUTRIENTS IN A BIO-AVAILABLE FORM, SO THAT A SIGNIFICANT PROPORTION CAN BE ABSORBED BY THE BODY.

This is especially true of nutrients such as zinc, iodine and folic acid, which play a crucial role in cell division in the body (which is when the errors that cause cancer are most likely to arise).

How?
● *Eat more fresh or lightly cooked vegetables and fruit, nuts and seeds, seaweed, fish and shellfish*
● *Have some brewers yeast and Icelandic kelp every day (follow the instructions on the packet or bottle and ensure you take the correct dose)*

5. REDUCE THE AMOUNT OF FREE RADICALS IN THE BODY WHICH ARE CAPABLE OF DAMAGING DNA.

How?
● *Yet more fruit and vegetables and whole grains*
● *Take a good quality selenium supplement*
● *Eat garlic, fresh herbs and spices*
● *Drink lots of green tea*

6. ELIMINATE OR REDUCE TO A MINIMUM FOOD THAT HAS BEEN REFINED, PRESERVED OR OVERCOOKED.

In such foods, the content of fibre, vitamins, minerals, natural colours or other natural constituents have been removed or reduced. Be especially vigilant in avoiding man-made chemical substances, including artificial vitamins or minerals.

How?
● *Cut out or cut down on manufactured convenience food especially anything with 'E' numbers in it. Frozen foods are usually OK and there is an increasing range of organically produced food available in bottles,*

jars and cans, which are fine occasionally
- *Cut down on or cut out refined sugar – use molasses, rice or maple syrup or honey*
- *Use brown unrefined flour, pasta and rice*
- *Ensure everything is as fresh, natural and as unaltered as possible*
- *Cut down on or cut out salt – use a little sea salt if absolutely necessary*
- *Substitute herbal teas such as camomile, fennel, peppermint, clover and green tea for black tea and coffee*
- *Do not drink alcohol, except for the occasional real ale, lager or quality organic wine*
- *Eat good freshly made food to avoid the need for vitamin or mineral supplements*

7. PROVIDE THE NUTRIENTS TO HELP YOUR BODY WITHSTAND AND RECOVER FROM SURGERY, RADIOTHERAPY AND CHEMOTHERAPY.

Many drugs, including those used in chemotherapy, destroy vitamins. Stress means you need more vitamins, while antibiotics can prevent them being absorbed.

How?
- *Eat unrefined food including wholegrain cereals*
- *Drink as much freshly made fruit and vegetable juice as possible*
- *Garlic, seaweed and organic eggs contain substances that help repair DNA*
- *Take brewer's yeast, which is a good source of B vitamins, folic acid and minerals*

8. PROVIDE MAXIMUM CHOICE AND VARIETY SO THAT HEALTHY EATING CAN BE MAINTAINED WITHOUT TOO MUCH RELIANCE ON ANY ONE FOOD SUBSTANCE.

How?
- *Have at least 30 different ingredients a day*
- *Use herbs and spices to add flavour*

All this might sound a bit daunting, but when you have adjusted and are preparing and eating the great meals described here, we believe you will be a convert for life – especially when your health and appearance begin to improve. Anyway, we have done all the hard work for you. All you need to do is make the delicious meals described and follow the simple point-scoring system to help prevent or treat breast or prostate cancer.

2.2 PRINCIPLES OF THE COOKBOOK

Many anti-cancer diets are difficult to keep to because the recipes are bland and boring and in some cases the regimes are harsh and extreme. Instead we have developed an exciting range of recipes based on the principles described in the previous section and inspired particularly by Asian cooking. Asian-style recipes often look complicated because they have a lot of ingredients, many of which are spices and herbs, but don't let this put you off. If you have a tray of all your spices to hand it is only about adding a few ingredients – it doesn't add a lot of time or make the dish complicated – it just adds flavour. Some anti-cancer diets eliminate all spices, although many spices, such as saffron, contain antioxidants and substances like circumin (in turmeric) have anti-cancer properties. Thai people have the lowest rates of breast and prostate cancer on record and Thai food is certainly spicy. The Avureydic medical system which has been used for centuries in India, also uses many spices.

The style of cooking used here ensures fresh, wholesome ingredients are cooked in the healthiest way possible and served while everything is still fresh. Two very important rules are:

● *Never use a microwave cooker, because free radicals are formed in the food*
● *Never use a pressure cooker, because it destroys vitamins and other important nutrients*

The style of cooking encourages social interaction. People today do not want to be relegated to the kitchen away from families and friends. The recipes that follow are based on a modern style of living, kitchens are open plan and everyone is encouraged to join in, chat to the cook and have a drink – in moderation, of course. Once you have adapted to asking a partner or friend to chop this or that, or encouraged your children to add something to the pan, you will enjoy cooking in a more open sociable environment. You will relax because everyone has played a part in creating the meal, even if it is just by chatting to the cook.

CUSTOMISING THE RECIPES

All the recipes contain a full list of ingredients, but we recommend you use them only as a guide and add or subtract ingredients to develop the meals that you enjoy the most.

Remember:
● *Any vegetable can be replaced with others. Use your favourite, what is in season or what is in the fridge. For example, change asparagus for beans and vice versa*
● *Although the recipes are based on measured quantities there are no hard and fast rules. Use what is left in a packet, or omit ingredients if you do not like their taste. You can do this without significantly changing the recipe*
● *Herbs and spices are a matter of preference, so vary the amounts according to your likes and dislikes. If you like spicy food we think you will enjoy the recipes as presented, but if you like milder food, simply cut down on the amount of spices, particularly chilli*
● *If you are on chemotherapy you may wish to reduce the amount of spices in the recipes. Replace them with extra fresh herbs*

The book includes a comprehensive set of recipes. In addition, the meals that you enjoy now may meet the principles of the programme or be adapted easily. Here are some simple changes to help you to make your usual meals healthier:

● *According to those great cooks Claudia Roden and Marcella Hazan, 'it is quite possible to substitute olive oil for butter in almost any dish'*
● *Soya 'milk' or 'cream' can be substituted for dairy milk or cream in most recipes*
● *Solid vegetable oil or grapeseed oil can substitute for butter to make pastry or cakes*

There are scare stories being circulated about soya. Despite reading many scientific papers about soya, we can find no convincing evidence that it causes cancer. Indeed authorities, such as the Royal Society, conclude that the phytoestrogens contained in soya are protective against breast and prostate cancer. Phytoestrogens are common in many foods from berries to whole grains, nuts and peas and beans.

USING YOUR LOCAL FARM SHOP OR ORGANIC FOOD SUPPLIER IS HELPING LOCAL INDUSTRY, REDUCING TRANSPORT-RELATED OUTPUT OF GREENHOUSE GASES, AND DOING YOUR BIT FOR THE ENVIRONMENT, AS WELL AS FOR YOURSELF

In order to help you to begin, the recipes have been organised into suggestions for breakfasts, snack and lunches or meals on the run and main meals. But most of the meals taste just as good at other times of the day. For example, most of the egg dishes are included in the breakfast section, but a delicious spicy vegetable omelette makes a quick and easy lunch served with a crisp salad, or served with other delicious dishes it can be included in a dinner menu. Similarly the soups described in the 'Meals on the run' section could be a full meal, a starter for dinner, or even a different breakfast.

To give you maximum flexibility in selecting your meals, we include a simple point-scoring system to encourage you to eat lots of raw fresh vegetables and fruit and to eat only moderate amounts of food from animal sources. Hence, a pear, artichoke and walnut, or any other meat-free salad, would score 0, so you can eat as much as you like, whenever you like. On the other hand, the barbecued lamb scores 10, so it is still OK in a cancer- prevention diet for special occasions, but we do not recommend you eat large quantities regularly.

SCORING SYSTEM
TYPE OF MEAL─CORE
- Fresh fruit and vegetable juices and salads   0
- Soya 'milk' and 'yoghurt', nuts, dried fruits, uncooked grains and bean curd (tofu)   1

- Mixed cooked and raw vegetables and fruit 2
- Cooked vegetables, fruit, grains and cooked dried pulses 3
- Canned beans, vegetables, soya 'cream' 4
- Dominantly vegetables with eggs 5
- Dominantly vegetables, with chicken, duck, fish and seafood 6
- Dominantly vegetables, with lamb, pork, rabbit, venison 7
- Dominantly egg 8
- Dominantly chicken, duck, fish and seafood 9
- Dominantly lamb, pork, rabbit or venison 10

The score for each recipe is shown in brackets after each recipe title.

PROGRAMME 1
Those with active cancer should not have any meal scoring more than 4, and they should aim for a daily score of around 15 to 20; but this can be averaged over the week to allow for an occasional treat.

PROGRAMME 2
Those on a prevention or maintenance programme should have a meal scoring more than 5 only once a day and should aim for a daily score of around 30 to 35, but this can be averaged over the week to allow for an occasional treat. This is the programme that Jane has followed for the past seven and a half years. She changed from programme 1 to programme 2 six months after her chemotherapy ended, and ten months after her cancer disappeared.

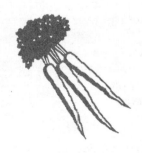

3 Dining In

WHAT YOU NEED

3.1 ESSENTIAL EQUIPMENT

We are assuming you have the usual range of cooking utensils, pots and pans, spoons, knives, etc. Here are some things you may not have, that you will need to make the recipes described here easier to prepare.

PREPARATION

● *FOOD PROCESSOR – there are many to choose from, the two most essential functions to look for are chopping and puréeing*
● *GRATERS OF DIFFERENT SIZES – to grate carrots, lemon peel, potatoes*
● *ICE CREAM MAKER (optional) – all of the sorbets and ice creams in this book have been made with a hand-turned ice cream maker with a metal freezer bowl, which is kept in the freezer.*
● *JUICER AND CITRUS SQUEEZER*
● *METAL PAN SCRUBBER – to scrub potatoes and root vegetables*
● *METRIC MEASURING CUPS AND SPOONS – will make it easier to follow the recipes*
● *MINCER (optional) – if you want to mince your own ingredients this is a very useful piece of equipment. Ours have a citrus squeezer and different-sized graters as attachments, and we use them regularly*
● *HAND-HELD BLENDER AND FOOD PROCESSOR ATTACHMENT – we find this the most useful piece of equipment in the kitchen. It is really great for chopping herbs, nuts, garlic, blending soups, making pastes, etc.*
● *SIEVES – to rinse rice and strain soups*
● *SALAD SHAKER – to ensure you dry salad vegetables thoroughly and do not water down the dressing.*

COOKING UTENSILS

● *CHARGRILL PAN – a ridged, flat frying pan that is a quick and easy alternative to a barbecue. Perfect for searing tuna or squid and cooking bacon*

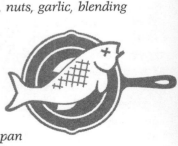

- *PEPPER AND SALT MILLS*
- *SAUTÉ PAN WITH LID – a wok can be used instead, but this is a very useful addition to your equipment*
- *STEAMER WITH LID (bamboo or stainless steel) – these come in a variety of sizes and are inexpensive in Asian food shops. They sit on top of a saucepan*
- *WOK – we use a non-stick finished wok with a lid. It is an essential piece of equipment for stir-frying vegetables and is a very versatile implement*

OTHER ESSENTIALS
- *GREASEPROOF PAPER*
- *BROWN PAPER BAGS*
- *ALUMINIUM FOIL*
- *STONE, GLASS OR EARTHENWARE STORAGE JARS*
- *WATER FILTER – GLASS JUG*

3.2 CLEARING THE DECKS AND RESTOCKING

- *Fresh is Best*
- *Frozen is Fine*
- *Herbs and spices add taste*
- *Organic for health*
- *Dump the dairy*

Most of the ingredients used in the recipes in this book are now readily available from supermarkets, but better still, enjoy searching out Asian shops, farmer and street markets, organic food and health shops and farm shops or farm suppliers. The Internet can help you to find fresh organic food locally, often with a free delivery service which is particularly helpful for those who are sick. Fooduk.com is the biggest UK outlet, but use search engines to find others. It is best to buy fresh food in season, because it is more nutritious, tastier and often cheaper.

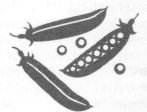

CLEARING THE DECKS

These are products we suggest you clear out of your home and your mind. If you have active cancer, **there are no half measures**. There is no point in having lots of good foods, while continuing to eat dairy products and junk food. So throw away:

● *MILK – from cows, sheep, goats, or any other animal; whether it is organic, skimmed, or semi-skimmed*

● *CHEESE – including so-called vegetarian cheese and cottage cheese*

● *YOGHURT – any kind (If you have had chemotherapy or a stomach infection, and need the good acidophilus bacteria, then have it in capsule form from your pharmacy. Just empty the contents of the gelatine capsule into a glass of soya 'milk' or water)*

● *CRÈME FRAÎCHE*

● *FROMAGE FRAIS*

● *CREAM*

● *BUTTER*

● *WHEY, LACTOSE, MILK SOLIDS, MILK FATS or CASEIN – these are often contained in processed or packaged foods*

● *MARGARINE*

● *BEEF or PORK MEATS – including processed meats, such as pâté, on the principle of not eating anything where you cannot identify the origin and ingredients*

● *COMMERCIAL REFINED AND PROCESSED OILS prepared using high pressure or temperature – including unspecified vegetable oils (which may contain genetically modified soya), maize oil, canola or rapeseed oil, or any products containing such oils*

● *SALT, REFINED WHITE FLOUR OR RICE, OTHER REFINED SUBSTANCES (such as aspartame), white sugar, or any foods containing these products (such as white bread and some pastas that have been chemically altered or depleted of fibre and nutrients)*

● *PROCESSED FOODS THAT CONTAIN **ANY** PRESERVATIVES – this **may** include such items as pre-packaged cookies, candies, cakes, crisps, soups, salted or spiced nuts, as well as processed meats (packaged hams, corned beef), bottled pickles, canned/cartoned fruit juices, and fruit drinks (always check the list of ingredients)*

● *COLOURED/FLAVOURED FIZZY DRINKS*

● *QUALITY or ORGANIC WINES AND SPIRITS can be taken in moderation, **except if you have active cancer**.*

THE RESTOCKED CUPBOARD

Here is a shopping list for the Plant Programme. It includes everything you will need for the recipes, as well as lots of other basics you may want to have in your cupboard (but it is not comprehensive). We have included some pre-prepared items, but be sure to check the ingredients carefully, and avoid those containing dairy products or preservatives. White bread can contain milk powder, and Indian bread or naan can contain yoghurt. Many commercial soups contain milk solids, and even vegetable soup can be in a whey base. The Jewish and oriental sections of supermarkets are often good sources of dairy-free products. Check against the list of forbidden dairy products in 'Clearing the decks'. If in doubt, ask the shop-owner or manager and do not allow yourself to be bluffed. **Dairy products are dairy products**, even when combined with other ingredients and processed. **Pure** vegetable 'milks' or 'butters', such as soya 'milk', cocoa or peanut butter, on the ingredient list are fine.

REMEMBER TO CHECK CAREFULLY FOR
'HIDDEN DAIRY' CASEIN, LACTOSE, WHEY

SHOPPING LIST

NON-DAIRY 'MILK', 'CREAM', 'YOGHURT' AND SPREADS
Coconut milk
Coconut cream
Peanut butter
Rice, oat or pea milk
Soya 'milk', 'cream' and 'yoghurt'
Soya spread

COOKING OILS, SAUCES AND STOCKS
Balsamic vinegar
Chicken, vegetable and fish stock cubes
Cider vinegar
Extra virgin olive oil
Fish sauce
Grapeseed oil
Light soya sauce

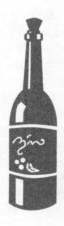

Oyster sauce
Peanut oil
Red wine vinegar
Sesame oil
Soya sauce
Sunflower oil
Thai fish sauce
Walnut oil
White wine vinegar

NUTS, GRAINS AND PULSES

Arborio rice
Basmati long grain rice
Cannellini beans
Chickpeas (dried or canned)
Cous cous
Egg noodles
Lentils
Nuts such as:
   cashew
   hazel
   macadamia
   peanut
   pistachio
   walnut
   (except Brazil – Brazil nuts can concentrate the radioactive
   element radium)

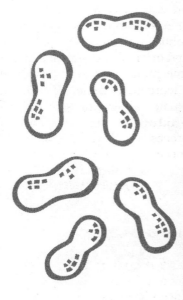

Oats and oat cakes
Pasta (all types)
Polenta
Red kidney beans (dried or canned)
Rice cakes
Rice noodles
Rice vermicelli noodles
Strong flour
Water chestnuts (bottled or canned standbys)
Wholemeal and rye breads
Wholemeal flour

BUY ORGANIC WHENEVER POSSIBLE

HERBS, SPICES AND SEASONINGS
FRESH
All herbs and spices including:
  Basil
  Bay leaves
  Chives
  Coriander
  Green chillies
  Italian parsley
  Lemon grass
  Lime leaves
  Mint
  Parsley
  Red chillies
  Thai basil

DRY
Bay leaves
Black pepper
Cayenne or chilli pepper
Cloves
Curry leaves
Garam masala
Ground cardamom
Ground cinnamon
Ground coriander
Ground cumin
Nutmeg
Sea salt
Tamarind
Turmeric

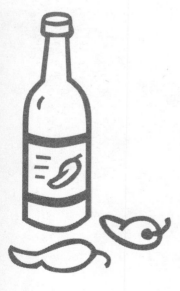

BOTTLED/CANNED
Capers
Chilli sauce
Green curry paste

EVEN IF YOU HAVE ONLY A WINDOW LEDGE,
YOU CAN GROW A VARIETY OF FRESH HERBS IN POTS.
THEY LOOK ATTRACTIVE AND ADD GREAT
FLAVOUR TO MEALS.

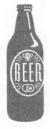

DRINKS
Herb teas
Green tea
Home-brewed beer
Real ale and lager
Cider
Pure cocoa

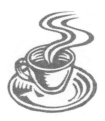

ALL FRESH HERBS/SPICES INCLUDING CHILLIES,
LIME LEAVES, GARLIC AND GINGER CAN BE FROZEN.
WRAP IN FOIL AND KEEP IN THE FREEZER.

FRUIT
Any fruit
Frozen fruit, without added sugar
Any dried fruit
Apricots
Dates
Figs
Raisins
Sultanas

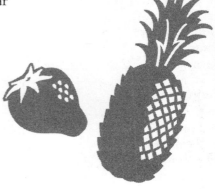

VEGETABLES
Any fresh vegetables, including:
Brown and red onions
Garlic
Ginger
Potatoes
Red, green, orange and yellow vegetables
Shallots
Sunblush tomatoes
Frozen vegetables
Frozen broad beans
Frozen corn

Frozen peas
Canned vegetables
Bamboo shoots
Italian tomatoes
Water chestnuts
Dried mushrooms
Marinated artichokes

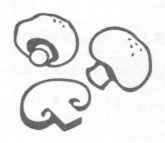

POULTRY, FISH & OTHER CORE INGREDIENTS
Lamb
Chicken
Duck
Rabbit
Venison/kangaroo/ostrich
Any ocean fish, except farmed fish (such as some salmon)
Small quantities of fresh water fish and shellfish
Smoked fish
All seafood
Eggs
Tofu, beancurd, tempeh, etc.
Any type of miso
Hummus
Taramasalata
Bacon or pork, from any rare breed of pig

SWEETENERS
Honey
Molasses
Raw cane sugar
Rice or maple syrup

PREPARED FOODS
Jams – look for those with the highest fruit concentrations,
    preferably sweetened with concentrated fruit juice
Bread – wholemeal; rye; some speciality breads
Biscuits – crispbread; rice crackers; some from the Chinese or
    Jewish sections of supermarkets
Chocolate – dark, dairy free

3.3 STORING FOOD

● *Fruit and vegetables should be eaten as soon as possible after harvesting. Buy small quantities frequently and store in the refrigerator*
● *Never store chopped or minced onion or garlic (it goes sour)*
● *Eggs, meat and fish should be stored in the refrigerator and eaten when quite fresh*
● *Grains and pulses, nuts, flour, pasta and spices can be stored in airtight glass or pottery storage jars at cool 'pantry' temperatures for weeks*
● *Oils need special care to avoid them going rancid. Unrefined or extra virgin oils will keep for up to six months if stored correctly. Keep them in dark stoppered glass bottles in dark cupboards at low 'pantry' temperatures*
● *Never store any food items in plastic – especially soft plastic. Use paper or aluminium foil or glass, metal or pottery containers instead.*

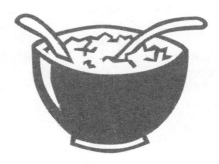

3.4 PREPARING FOOD

● *Fruit and vegetables should be washed thoroughly and peeled if they are not organic*
● *Do not cut fruit and vegetables before washing*
● *Dip organic produce, which is to be eaten raw, in boiling water (this is especially important if your immunity is impaired)*
● *Scrub potatoes and other root vegetables with a metal pan scrubber. This will remove dirt and germs, but preserve more nutrients than peeling*

● *Use a salad shaker to remove excess water from salad vegetables. Then pat them dry using a clean cloth or unbleached kitchen paper*
● *Leave washed fruit and vegetables, other than salad vegetables, to drain in a colander before drying with a clean cloth or unbleached kitchen paper*
● *Keep fresh lemon juice to hand to stop chopped apple, pear or avocado turning brown*
● *Never store juices*
● *Wash meat and fish thoroughly and pat dry before cooking*
● *Wash rice, lentils, dried beans and peas in a sieve under running water. Look out for small stones especially in lentils*
● *Dried beans and peas need soaking before cooking. Put them in the pan they will be cooked in. Cover with filtered water in the proportion of 4 cups of water to one cup of beans. Leave to stand for 8 hours or overnight (split peas need only 3 hours). Alternatively, bring the beans and water to the boil and cook for 2 minutes before leaving them to stand for 1 hour. Cook in the water used for soaking for approximately 2 hours*
● *Lentils can be cooked without soaking*
● *Soak and pre-cook large quantities of beans and peas and freeze them. Frozen cooked beans are almost as convenient to use as canned ones. Add them directly to soups and casseroles.*

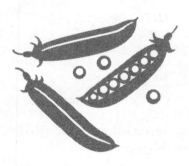

4 Food for the week

DAILY/WEEKLY MENU PLANS

4.1 FOR THOSE WITH ACTIVE CANCER

- *Lots of fresh fruit and vegetable juices*
- *A melon juice every day*
- *At least one raw vegetable salad every day*
- *2–3 pieces of fresh fruit every day*
- *One serving of rice or grain every day*
- *Lots of fibre*
- *More herbs than spice*
- *A very occasional egg, fish, chicken or prawn dish*
- *No caffeine or alcohol other than the occasional beer*
- *Herbal teas and filtered boiled water*
- *Lots of green tea*

If you are undergoing chemotherapy, you probably will not feel like eating for a day or so after your treatment. However, the sooner you can eat some tempting nutritious food the better. Here are some examples of menus which are suitable for those with active breast or prostate cancer.

REMEMBER TO DISCUSS YOUR CHANGE OF DIET WITH YOUR ONCOLOGIST, GENERAL PRACTITIONER OR PHYSICIAN.

MONDAY
BREAKFAST
Tomato, celery and carrot juice (page 39–40)   (0)
Cereal with soya milk' sprinkled with chopped linseed,
   sunflower and almonds (page 43)   (2)

MID MORNING
Watermelon and blueberry juice   (0)

LUNCH
Asian vegetable salad (page 82–3)   (0)
Fresh fruit   (0)

MID AFTERNOON
Peppermint, camomile, fennel or nettle tea

DINNER
Sweet potato and coconut soup (page 75–6)   (3)
Stirfried bean-curd with snowpeas and steamed rice (page 140) (3)
Marinated oranges with chocolate sorbet (pages 207–8 and 202) (0)

PRE BEDTIME
Pineapple and apple juice

DAILY SCORE: 11 / NO OF INGREDIENTS: 39*

TUESDAY
BREAKFAST
Fennel, celery and carrot juice (page 39–40)   (0)
Potato, avocado and tomato stacks (leave out the bacon)
(page 53–4)   (2)

MID MORNING
Apple and kiwifruit juice   (0)

LUNCH
Tomato and avocado bruschetta (page 109)   (3)
Thai salad (page 94–5)   (0)

MID AFTERNOON
Peppermint, camomile, fennel or nettle tea

DINNER
Carrot and orange soup (page 65–6)   (3)
Chickpeas with roasted vegetables   (3)
Strawberries in balsamic vinegar   (0)

PRE BEDTIME
Banana smoothie (page 222)   (1)

DAILY SCORE: 12 / NO OF INGREDIENTS: 43

WEDNESDAY
BREAKFAST
Carrot and orange juice (page 40)   (0)
Hummus on toast (page 107)   (3)

MID MORNING
Fennel, celery and green apple   (0)

LUNCH
Red lentil salad (page 148–9)   (3)
Fresh fruit   (0)

MID AFTERNOON
Peppermint, camomile, fennel or nettle tea

DINNER
Spinach soup (page 74)   (3)
Fried rice (page 126)   (3)
Tropical fruit salad (page 41–2)(0) with nut 'cream' (page 210)   (1)

PRE BEDTIME
Chocolate soya 'milk' (page 224–5)   (1)

DAILY SCORE: 14 / NO OF INGREDIENTS: 46

THURSDAY
BREAKFAST
Mango and apple juice   (0)
Rice porridge with coconut milk (page 44–5)   (3)

MID MORNING
Red pepper, carrot and lettuce juice   (0)

LUNCH
Nicoise salad (no chicken) (page 99)   (0)
Fresh fruit   (0)

MID AFTERNOON
Peppermint, camomile, fennel or nettle tea

DINNER
Cauliflower and potato curry (page 150)   (3)
Stir-fried fennel and bok choy (page 156)   (0)
Steamed rice   (3)
Banana ice cream (page 202)   (4)

PRE BEDTIME
Cucumber and kiwifruit   (0)

DAILY SCORE: 13 / NO OF INGREDIENTS: 41

FRIDAY
BREAKFAST
Strawberry and pear juice   (0)
Grilled mushrooms on toast (page 51)   (3)

MID MORNING
Carrot, cucumber, spinach and green pepper juice   (0)

LUNCH
Baked potato with dip of choice   (3)
Carrot salad (page 85)   (1)
Green bean salad (page 100)   (3)

MID AFTERNOON
Peppermint, camomile, fennel or nettle tea

DINNER
Red pepper soup (page 72–3)   (3)
Tomato and olive pizza (page 229–31)   (3)
Fresh fruit   (0)

PRE BEDTIME
Apple and celery juice (0)

DAILY SCORE: 16 / NO OF INGREDIENTS: 38

SATURDAY
BREAKFAST
Mixed berry fruit salad (0) with soya 'yoghurt' (1)
Toast with spread of choice (3)

MID MORNING
Carrot and orange juice (0)

LUNCH
Pear, walnut and artichoke salad (page 90) (0)
Olive bread (page 60) (3)

MID AFTERNOON
Peppermint, camomile, fennel or nettle tea

DINNER
Tomato soup (page 77) (3)
Penne with green vegetables (page 117) (3)
Fresh fruit (0)

PRE BEDTIME
Chocolate soya 'milk' (1)

DAILY SCORE: 14 / NO OF INGREDIENTS: 40

SUNDAY
BREAKFAST
Tomato, celery and carrot juice (0)
Rice with lentils (page 55) (3)

MID MORNING
Apple and mango juice (0)

LUNCH
Onion and garlic soup (page 71)   (3)
Chickpeas with roasted pumpkin and sweet potato (page 144–5) (3)
Green salad with coconut dressing (page 86–7)   (4)
Banana with chocolate sorbet (page 202)   (0)

MID AFTERNOON
Peppermint, camomile, fennel or nettle tea

DINNER
Baked potato with dip of choice   (3)
Red onion and tomato salsa (page 91–2)   (0)
Avocado and papaya salad (page 83)   (0)

PRE BEDTIME
Fennel and kiwifruit juice   (0)

DAILY SCORE: 15 / NO OF INGREDIENTS: 55

4.2 FOR THOSE ON A PREVENTION OR MAINTENANCE DIET

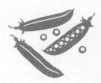

- ● *Plenty of variety*
- ● *Fruit and vegetable juices*
- ● *Animal protein maximum once a day to comprise less than 25% of meal*
- ● *One raw vegetable salad per day*
- ● *Spices and herbs for taste*

We have assumed a working person's lifestyle, with the main meal of the day in the evening during the week, and a more leisurely breakfast or brunch at the weekend, and a family lunch on Sunday. The menus can be adapted simply to your own needs.

MONDAY
BREAKFAST
Grapefruit, kiwi and red grape juice   (0)

Potato, avocado and tomato stacks (page 53-4) (7)
  (use left-over potatoes)

MID MORNING
Peppermint, camomile, fennel or nettle tea

LUNCH
Rice salad (page 92–3) (3)
Carrot salad (page 85) (1)
Fresh fruit (0)

PRE-DINNER
Carrot and orange juice (0)

DINNER
Chicken and coconut milk soup (page 66) (6)
Bean curd with snowpeas and red pepper (page 140) (3)
Marinated oranges with nut 'cream' (pages 207–8 and 210) (1)

DAILY SCORE: 21 / NO OF INGREDIENTS: 42

TUESDAY
BREAKFAST
Orange, grapefruit and cranberry juice (0)
Scrambled eggs with tomato and mushroom (page 48) (8)

MID MORNING
Peppermint, camomile, fennel or nettle tea

LUNCH
Pear, walnut and artichoke salad (page 90) (0)

PRE-DINNER
Tomato, celery and carrot juice (page 39–40) (0)

DINNER
Cauliflower and potato curry (page 150) (3)
Stir-fried fennel and bok choy (page 156) (3)

Steamed rice	(3)
Pineapple slices with kirsch and chocolate sauce	(0)

DAILY SCORE: 17 / NO OF INGREDIENTS: 35

WEDNESDAY
BREAKFAST

Watermelon, blueberries, ginger and basil juice	(0)
Grilled mushrooms on toast (page 51)	(3)

MID MORNING
Peppermint, camomile, fennel or nettle tea

LUNCH

Mixed green salad (page 88–9)	(0)
Carrot salad (page 85)	(1)
Fresh bread	(3)
Fresh fruit	(0)

PRE-DINNER

Alfalfa and carrot juice	(0)

DINNER

Sweet potato soup (page 75–6)	(4)
Duck and melon salad (page 98)	(6)
Spicy potatoes (page 154–5)	(3)
Strawberries in balsamic vinegar (0) with soya 'cream'	(4)

DAILY SCORE: 21 / NO OF INGREDIENTS: 46

THURSDAY
BREAKFAST

Apple and strawberry juice	(0)
Cereal sprinkled with linseed, sunflower and almond mix with soya 'milk' (page 43)	(1)

MID MORNING
Peppermint, camomile, fennel or nettle tea

LUNCH
Avocado and tomato sandwich (page 104)   (3)
Fresh fruit   (0)

PRE-DINNER
Apple and celery juice   (0)

DINNER
Red pepper soup (page 72–3)   (3)
Flaked fish in lettuce leaves (page 174)   (9)
Thai-style green salad (page 94–5)   (0)
Mango in Bacardi   (0)

DAILY SCORE: 16 / NO OF INGREDIENTS: 36

FRIDAY
BREAKFAST
Melon and raspberry juice   (0)
Tomato bruschetta (page 109)   (3)

MID MORNING
Peppermint, camomile, fennel or nettle tea

LUNCH
Prawn and beansprout salad   (6)
Fresh fruit   (0)

PRE-DINNER
Fennel, celery and green apple juice   (0)

DINNER
Stuffed aubergine (page 160)   (3)
Fish stew (page 170–1)   (9)
Banana in coconut custard   (4)

DAILY SCORE: 25 / NO OF INGREDIENTS: 47

SATURDAY
BREAKFAST
Pineapple with coconut milk (page 39)   (4)
Kedgeree (page 54–5)   (6)

MID MORNING
Peppermint, camomile, fennel or nettle tea

LUNCH
Baked potato and dip of choice   (3)
Mixed green salad (page 88–9)   (0)
Fresh fruit   (0)

PRE-DINNER
Red pepper, carrot and lettuce juice   (0)

DINNER
Tomato soup (page 77)   (3)
Paella (page 128)   (6)
Mandarin sorbet (page 203)   (0)

DAILY SCORE: 22 / NO OF INGREDIENTS: 46

SUNDAY

BREAKFAST
Spicy tomato, cucumber and carrot juice (0)
  (with vodka optional)
Crab omelette (page 46) (8)

MID MORNING
Peppermint, camomile, fennel or nettle tea

LUNCH
Roast chicken with lemons (page 184–5) (9)
Green beans with garlic (page 152) (3)
Mixed green salad (page 88–9) (0)
Baby roast potatoes with rosemary and garlic (3)
Apple crumble (3)

PRE-DINNER
Carrot cake (page 215) (3)
Herbal tea

DINNER
Minted pea and potato soup (page 69) (3)
Fresh bread (3)

DAILY SCORE: 35 / NO OF INGREDIENTS: 39

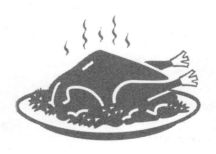

4.3 DINNER PARTY MENUS

1

Simple mulligatawny soup

Barbecued spiced leg of lamb
Spicy cumin potatoes
Green beans with garlic
Red onion and tomato salsa

Mandarin sorbet
Pecan biscuits

2

Vegetable samosas

Lamb with green peppers
Vegetables in coconut milk
Dhal (spicy chickpeas)
Plain rice

Coconut crème caramel

3

Spinach soup

Green curry chicken
Stir-fried Asian vegetables
Steamed rice

Tropical fruit salad
with coconut ice cream

4

Carrot, beetroot, aubergine
and hummus dips
Marinated mushrooms
Zucchini in red wine vinegar
Olives
Pitta bread

Roast lamb
Chickpeas with roasted
vegetables

Orange and almond cake

5

Gazpacho soup

Paella

Fresh fruit salad
and nut 'cream'

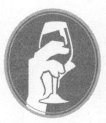

5 Good beginnings

- *Freshly squeezed vegetable or fruit juice*
- *Lots of fresh fruit*
- *Honey or molasses or raw cane muscovado sugar instead of refined white sugar*
- *Muesli, porridge, rice, noodles*
- *Occasional eggs or fish*
- *Soya, coconut, rice or oat 'milk', instead of dairy milk*
- *Soya 'yoghurt' and 'cream', instead of dairy yoghurt or cream*

Breakfasts are very much a matter of personal preference. Some people prefer only a light meal while for others breakfast is the most important meal of the day. Some of the best breakfasts are very simple. If you prefer a full traditional British- or Irish-style breakfast, such as egg, bacon, mushrooms, tomatoes (but **not** commercial sausages), or kippers, go ahead – as long as you grill or cook with olive oil or pure soya spread and limit the bacon. Such a meal scores between 5 and 10, depending on the amount of food from animal sources. If you have active cancer, leave out the bacon and kippers, and limit the amount of egg.

If you want to be more adventurous here are some new ideas, including some Asian dishes to make your breakfast time more exciting.

5.1 JUICES TO START THE DAY

We recommend that everyone starts the day with a glass of freshly made fruit and/or vegetable juice.

Most combinations of fruit and vegetable juice are tasty and healthy. Here are some of our favourites, but do experiment and invent some of your own, bearing in mind that onions and a few other vegetables, such as watercress, have a very strong flavour, so use just a little.

- *Don't have too much raw cabbage juice, because it can cause problems with the thyroid*
- *Don't have too much carrot juice, as it can make you turn orange*

(both of us have a limit of about one cup a day)

● Don't have too many acid fruits and vegetables such as citrus fruits, berries, tomatoes and beetroot, especially if you are on chemotherapy or have aching joints or muscles.

Fresh juices should be drunk immediately to ensure that the precious vitamins and other active components are not lost on contact with air (you can see how quickly apple juice goes brown) – so don't make large quantities to store in the fridge. Instead, keep your juicer close at hand on your workbench rather than at the back of a cupboard.

If you keep your fruit in the fridge the juice will be nicely chilled. Alternatively, chill juices by adding ice cubes or crushed ice.

WASH ALL YOUR FRUIT AND VEGETABLES THOROUGHLY BEFORE JUICING, AND PEEL THEM UNLESS YOU ARE SURE THE FRUIT IS UNWAXED.

● Soft fruits such as bananas, peaches, apricots, melons, papaya (paw paw), mango, strawberries and other berries should be processed in a blender. Mix with

other fruit juices or just dilute with some filtered water or blend with soya 'milk'

● Squeeze citrus fruits in a citrus press

● Use a juicer for all other fruits and vegetables.

FRESH WATERMELON JUICE (0)

Watermelon is especially rich in folic acid which helps cells divide correctly and helps to prevent hair loss with some types of chemotherapy.

CORE INGREDIENT
1/2 medium watermelon

1 Cut the watermelon into large chunks, after removing the skin. Put it into a food processor or blender, pips and all, and purée. It couldn't be simpler.

PREPARATION TIME:
1–2 minutes

FRUIT JUICE SUGGESTIONS (0)

● 1 kiwifruit, 1/2 grapefruit and 1 cup red seedless grapes
● 1 cup watermelon, 1/2 cup blueberries, (mixed with 1 tsp minced fresh ginger and 5–6 shredded basil leaves)
● 1/2 melon with 1 cup raspberries
● 2 kiwifruit with 2 pears

● *1 mango with 1/4 cup*
lemon juice
● *mango and apricot or peach*
diluted with water
● *2 apples or pears and 1 mango*
● *2 apples and 2 pears*
● *2 apples, 3-4 celery sticks*
(with leaves) and 1/2 lemon
● *2 nectarines, 12 red grapes*
and 1 kiwifruit
● *2 apples or pears and 1 cup*
strawberries
● *1 small orange, 1/2 grapefruit*
and 1/2 cup cranberries
● *1/2 pineapple and 2 apples.*

These quantities all make about
1 cup of juice.

GREEN BRAMLEY
COOKING APPLES ARE
THE BEST FOR JUICING
AND CONTAIN LOTS OF
VITAMIN C AND FOLIC
ACID. CRISP GRANNY
SMITHS ARE ALSO
DELICIOUS JUICED.
IF YOU KNOW THEY
ARE ORGANIC, THEN
DO NOT BOTHER
TO PEEL THEM.
NEVER USE SOFT OR
RED SKINNED APPLES.

FRESH PINEAPPLE WITH COCONUT MILK (4)
CORE INGREDIENT
1/2 fresh pineapple, peeled
  and cored

FROM THE CUPBOARD
1/2 cup coconut milk

1 Mix the pineapple and
coconut milk in a blender and
process until smooth. Add some
crushed ice and serve. Dilute
with a little water if necessary.

PREPARATION TIME:
3-4 minutes

TOMATO, CELERY AND CARROT JUICE (0)
CORE INGREDIENT
2 medium–large tomatoes

FRUIT/VEGETABLES
2-3 sticks of celery
1 carrot
1/2 medium fennel bulb
1 clove of garlic
1/2 T lemon juice

HERBS AND SPICES
salt and pepper to taste
a few drops of Tabasco sauce
1/2 tsp of Worcestershire sauce

1 Wash and trim the vegetables,
cut into coarse chunks and
process through the juicer

2 Serve with lemon juice, salt and pepper, and add Tabasco and Worcestershire sauce to taste.

PREPARATION TIME:
2–3 minutes

VEGETABLE JUICE SUGGESTIONS (0)

● *2 carrots, 1 large orange*
● *100 gm alfalfa, 3 carrots*
● *125 gm kale, 2 carrots, 1/2 red pepper*
● *2 carrots, 1 cup of spinach, 1/2 cucumber, 1/2 green pepper*
● *3 carrots, 1/2 beetroot, 1 apple*
● *1/2 cucumber, 2 kiwifruit*
● *1/2 small lettuce, 2 sticks of celery, 1 apple*
● *1 red pepper, 2 carrots, 1/2 small lettuce*
● *1/2 fennel bulb, 2 sticks celery, 1 green apple.*

These quantities all make about 1 cup of juice.

5.2 FRUIT TREATS

Fresh fruit is packed with vitamins, minerals and other anti-cancer chemicals and berries contain phytoestrogens. Eating fresh fruit is much better for you than popping vitamin supplements. You should aim to eat at least 2–3 pieces of fruit every day.

MIXED BERRY FRUIT SALAD (0) SERVED WITH SOYA 'YOGHURT' (1)

CORE INGREDIENT
500 gm mixed berries – strawberries, raspberries, blueberries, blackberries

FRUIT/VEGETABLES
juice of 1/2 an orange

FROM THE CUPBOARD
1 T sugar
250 ml plain or flavoured soya 'yoghurt'

1 Wash the fruit and drain thoroughly
2 Mix the fruit together gently in a serving bowl varying the proportions to taste
3 Pour over the orange juice, sprinkle with a little sugar to taste and serve with soya 'yoghurt'.

PREPARATION TIME:
2–3 minutes

FRESH FRUIT SUGGESTIONS (0)

● *Papaya served with fresh lime juice*
● *Rockmelon, honeydew melon, watermelon with sugar syrup, and finely chopped preserved ginger*

● *Honeydew melon and papaya with lemon juice*
● *Orange, apple, grapes, pitted lychees with fresh lime juice*
● *Kiwifruit, apple, strawberries, with fresh lemon juice*

PEACH AND STRAWBERRIES WITH PURÉED RASPBERRIES (0) AND FLAVOURED SOYABEAN CURD (1)

Flavoured soyabean is beginning to appear in the better health food shops. Coconut and mango flavours are especially delicious. Serve chilled.

CORE INGREDIENT
3 peaches, sliced

FRUIT/VEGETABLES
125 gm strawberries, sliced
125 gm raspberries
1 T lemon juice

FROM THE CUPBOARD
1 T cane sugar or honey
1/4 cup water
flavoured bean curd

1 Mix the strawberries and peaches together gently
2 Purée the raspberries in a food processor or blender with the lemon juice and a little sugar syrup to taste. (We prefer the raspberry purée without sugar)
3 Put the fruit into pretty bowls, pour over the raspberry purée and serve with flavoured soyabean curd.

The raspberry purée can be made with either fresh or thawed frozen raspberries.

PREPARATION TIME:
4–5 minutes

MAKE SUGAR SYRUP BY DISSOLVING SUGAR OR HONEY IN BOILING WATER. ADD ONE TEASPOON OF BALSAMIC VINEGAR TO UNDERRIPE OR TASTELESS STRAWBERRIES TO ENHANCE THEIR FLAVOUR.

TROPICAL FRUIT SALAD (0)

Use any combination of fruit, choose your favourites.

CORE INGREDIENT
500 gm mixed tropical fruits –
  1/2 papaya, 1/4 pineapple,
  2 kiwifruit, 8 lychees, 1/4
  watermelon, 1 banana,
  2 passion fruit

FRUIT/VEGETABLES
1–2 T lemon or lime juice

1 Wash, dry and prepare the fruit and mix together gently, or arrange separately on a plate, reserving the passion fruit
2 Cut the passion fruit in half and squeeze the pulp over the rest of the fruit
3 Drizzle the lemon or lime juice over the fruit, stir and serve.

PREPARATION TIME:
10 minutes

MANGO 'YOGHURT' (1)
CORE INGREDIENT
1 mango, skinned, seeded and cut into chunks

FROM THE CUPBOARD
200 gm plain soya 'yoghurt'
1–2 tsp honey (or to taste)
1/2 cup almonds or pine nuts

1 Purée the mango in a food processor
2 Toast the almonds or pine nuts in the oven or in a hot pan for a few minutes until they turn light brown
3 Mix the mango and soya 'yoghurt' together and add honey to taste
4 Sprinkle with toasted almonds or pine nuts and serve in breakfast bowls.

PREPARATION TIME:
6–8 minutes

VARIATION:
● *Use peaches, raspberries or any other soft fruit.*

POACHED DRIED FIGS (1)
CORE INGREDIENT
250 gm dried figs

FRUIT/VEGETABLES
'Zest' or grated peel of an orange
2 T orange juice

FROM THE CUPBOARD
1/2 cup sugar or 3 T honey
1 cup of water
1/2 cup of almonds or pine nuts
plain soya 'yoghurt'

HERBS AND SPICES
1 cinnamon stick

1 Boil the water and sugar or honey together on medium heat stirring until it dissolves to make a syrup
2 Add the orange juice, cinnamon, orange zest and figs, and simmer for about 20 minutes, then remove from the heat and allow to cool
3 Toast the almonds or pine nuts
4 Serve the figs with soya 'yoghurt' sprinkled with the toasted nuts.

PREPARATION TIME:
3–4 minutes/COOKING TIME:
25 minutes

VARIATIONS:
● *This dish can also be made with 8 fresh figs*
● *For a delicious dessert add brandy to the orange juice and serve with coconut milk*

FIGS CAN BE EATEN FRESH OR HEATED THROUGH UNDER A GRILL

5.3 SUBSTANTIAL STARTERS

A nutritious breakfast is a good start to the day especially if you are recovering from illness and the side effects of medical treatment.

GRAINS AND CEREALS

Bought breakfast cereals such as whole wheat, cereal bars and health store muesli are fine, but you can make your own delicious healthy alternatives, which can be stored in airtight jars for a week or so. Serve cereals with soya or coconut milk. Low-fat coconut milk, which is a healthy alternative, is now available. If you have difficulty with wheat, substitute other gluten-free cereals, such as oats or rice.

SOYA 'MILK' IS RICH IN CALCIUM. BEAN CURD OR TOFU IS MADE BY PRECIPITATING SOYA 'MILK' WITH CALCIUM OR MAGNESIUM SALTS.

LINSEED, SUNFLOWER SEED AND ALMOND MIX (1)

This is a healthy addition to any cereal, salad or dessert to provide essential fibre, vitamins and other nutrients including phytoestrogens.

CORE INGREDIENT
1 cup of linseed

FROM THE CUPBOARD
1 cup of almonds
1 cup of sunflower seeds

1 Put all the ingredients into a food processor or coffer grinder and process until finely chopped
2 Store in an airtight container, it will last for weeks.

PREPARATION TIME:
2–3 minutes

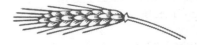

NUTS AND OATS (1)
CORE INGREDIENT
125gm toasted nuts

FROM THE CUPBOARD
200 gm dried fruit
200 gm toasted bran
200 gm toasted oat flakes
1 T poppy seeds
honey to taste

1 Mix all the dry ingredients together and store in an airtight container
2 Serve with fresh fruit of your choice, such as banana and soya 'yoghurt'. Alternatively, try fresh orange or apple juice
3 Sprinkle with the linseed, sunflower and almond mix (page 00)

PREPARATION TIME:
1–2 minutes

ORGANIC MUESLI (1)
CORE INGREDIENT
2 cups rolled oats

FRUIT/VEGETABLES
2 Granny Smith apples, grated
1 T lemon juice
1 cup fresh strawberries or raspberries or blueberries (optional)

FROM THE CUPBOARD
1 T honey

½ cup coarsely ground mixed nuts (almonds, walnuts, hazelnuts, etc.)
½ cup raisins
1 cup soya 'milk', water or orange juice
soya 'yoghurt' to serve

1 Soak the oats overnight in the water, orange juice, soya 'milk' or coconut milk
2 Drizzle the lemon juice over the apple and stir to stop the apple going brown
3 Add the nuts, apple and berries to the oats
4 Serve with additional soya 'milk' or orange juice and some soya 'yoghurt'.

PREPARATION TIME: 5 minutes, plus overnight soaking

RICE PORRIDGE WITH COCONUT MILK (4)
Gill's Australian husband swears that this is the best breakfast 'bush tucker'. He discovered it whilst working in northern Papua New Guinea in 1980.

CORE INGREDIENT
1 cup of short grained rice

FRUIT/VEGETABLES
2 bananas or 2 peaches, sliced (optional)

FROM THE CUPBOARD
2 cups of coconut milk
1/2 –1 cup of water
1/2 cup of slivered almonds
1/2 cup of raisins
2 T honey or maple syrup

HERBS AND SPICES
5–6 cardamom pods, crushed

1 Simmer the rice with the coconut milk, water, honey or syrup and the crushed cardamom pods. Stir frequently, until the rice is cooked (approximately 25 minutes). If the rice goes dry before it is cooked just add a little more water
2 Mix in the sliced almonds and raisins
3 Serve with peaches or bananas.

PREPARATION TIME:
1–2 minutes/COOKING TIME:
25–30 mins

DO NOT OVERCOOK OMELETTES OR THEY WILL GO RUBBERY. OMELETTES NEED TO BE COOKED ON BOTH SIDES; THE SIMPLEST WAY, ESPECIALLY IF THE OMELETTE CONTAINS COOKED VEGETABLES, IS TO COOK IT IN A FRYING PAN UNTIL THE UNDERSIDE IS DONE AND THEN FINISH OFF THE TOP UNDER A GRILL. ALTERNATIVELY, YOU CAN SLIDE THE OMELETTE ON TO A PLATE, PUT ANOTHER PLATE ON TOP, TURN AND SLIDE BACK INTO THE FRYING PAN; OR YOU CAN JUST FLIP THE OMELETTE OVER. WE FIND THE FIRST METHOD THE EASIEST.

5.4 EASY EGGS

Eggs are the ultimate fast food and are good boiled, poached, or scrambled with soya 'milk' and soya spread or even fried in olive oil, but there are many interesting and delicious variations to try.

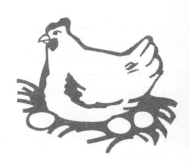

CRAB AND BEANSPROUT OMELETTE (8)

CORE INGREDIENT
4 eggs
125 gm crab meat

FRUIT/VEGETABLES
100 gm bean sprouts
4 spring onions, chopped

FROM THE CUPBOARD
1 T olive oil

HERBS AND SPICES
1 tsp chilli sauce (optional)
chopped coriander or parsley
  (optional)
salt and pepper to taste

1 Beat the eggs lightly
2 Fold in the crabmeat, bean sprouts and spring onions and season to taste
3 Heat the olive oil in a frying pan, pour in the egg mixture and cook until the underside of the omelette is cooked
4 Heat the grill and place the omelette under the heat until the top is cooked through
5 Serve with fresh parsley or for a more exotic flavour fresh coriander and chilli sauce.

PREPARATION TIME:
2–3 minutes/COOKING TIME:
4–5 minutes

INDONESIAN-STYLE FRIED RICE (NASI GORENG) (5)

This dish will surprise you! It is the Southeast Asian equivalent of the British breakfast, and it's very full and satisfying. Ideal for a weekend brunch.

CORE INGREDIENT
4 eggs

FRUIT/VEGETABLES
1 onion, chopped
4–5 cloves garlic, sliced
4 spring onions, chopped
1 cup of peas

FROM THE CUPBOARD
1–2 T olive oil
2 T light soya sauce
2 T water
2 1/2 cups of cooked basmati rice

HERBS AND SPICES
2 T fresh coriander
salt and pepper to taste
chilli sauce (optional)

1 Heat the oil and sauté the onion until it begins to turn brown. Add the garlic and fry for another minute
2 Add the rice, peas and spring onions and sauté for 2–3 minutes. Add the water and soya sauce, cover and continue cooking until the rice is heated through

3 In a separate pan, lightly fry or poach the eggs
4 Serve the rice on a plate and top with an egg and garnish with coriander. Serve with extra soya sauce and/or chilli sauce.

PREPARATION TIME: 5–6 mins
COOKING TIME: 6–8 mins

VARIATION:
● *Add red or green pepper or other vegetables of choice to the rice and omit the egg (3).*

MIXED VEGETABLE OMELETTE (5)
CORE INGREDIENT
4 eggs

FRUIT/VEGETABLES
1 onion, chopped
2 cloves garlic, finely chopped
1 cup of green beans, cut into 2 1/2 cm lengths
1/2 green pepper, seeded and chopped
1/2 red pepper, seeded and chopped
1 cup frozen peas
1 cup frozen corn

FROM THE CUPBOARD
1 T olive oil

HERBS AND SPICES
salt and pepper to taste
chopped chives and/or parsley

1 Heat the olive oil and fry the onion for 2 to 3 minutes. Add the garlic and fry for another minute
2 Add the green beans, the green and red peppers and continue cooking for about 4 minutes, then add the peas and corn and continue to cook until they are warmed through but still crunchy
3 Lightly beat the eggs then pour them over the vegetables and cook until the underside of the omelette is cooked
4 Heat the grill and place the pan under the heat until the top of the omelette is cooked through
5 Serve sprinkled with fresh chopped chives or parsley.

PREPARATION TIME:
10 minutes/COOKING TIME:
15 minutes

SAUTÉED SPINACH WITH POACHED EGGS (5)
CORE INGREDIENT
4 eggs

FRUIT/VEGETABLES
2–3 cloves garlic, chopped
500 gm fresh spinach

FROM THE CUPBOARD
1 T olive oil

HERBS AND SPICES
salt and pepper

1 Wash the spinach and
drain well
2 Poach the eggs in gently
simmering water until cooked
to your liking
3 Heat the olive oil, add the
garlic and cook for about 1
minute until it turns golden
4 Add the spinach and sauté for
1–2 minutes until it starts to wilt
5 Serve the spinach with the
poached egg on top and season
to taste.

PREPARATION TIME:
1–2 minutes/COOKING TIME:
3–4 minutes

ALTERNATIVE: Line ovenproof
dishes with the spinach leaves,
season with salt and pepper,
break the egg into the middle of
the spinach and bake in a
preheated 180°C oven until the
egg is cooked to your liking –
approximately 13 to 15 minutes.

VARIATION:
● *Serve poached egg over steamed
asparagus or green beans (5).*

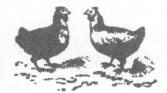

SCRAMBLED EGGS WITH TOMATO AND MUSHROOMS (8)

CORE INGREDIENT
4 eggs

FRUIT/VEGETABLES
4–5 cloves garlic, chopped
3 vine-ripened tomatoes, sliced
12 baby mushrooms, halved

FROM THE CUPBOARD
2 T olive oil
2 T water

HERBS AND SPICES
2 T parsley or basil
2 T chopped chives
salt and pepper to taste

1 Heat the olive oil, add the
garlic and fry until it begins to
change colour
2 Add the sliced tomato and
season to taste. Cook for 1 to 2
minutes on one side and then
turn the tomatoes over, add the
mushrooms and continue to
cook for another minute (do
not overcook the tomatoes)
3 Lightly beat the eggs with the
water and add to the tomatoes,
stir gently while cooking until
the egg sets to your liking
4 Serve sprinkled with chopped
herbs.

PREPARATION TIME:
1–2 minutes/COOKING TIME:
5–6 minutes

SPINACH OMELETTE (8)
CORE INGREDIENT
4 eggs

FRUIT/VEGETABLES
1 large onion, finely chopped
3–4 cloves garlic, minced
1 large tomato, chopped
250 gm fresh baby spinach
  leaves

FROM THE CUPBOARD
2 T olive oil

HERBS AND SPICES
salt and pepper
2 T chopped parsley or oregano
2 T chopped chives (optional)

1 Wash the spinach and drain
well
2 Heat the olive oil, add the
chopped onion and cook over a
medium heat until the onion
starts to turn translucent
3 Add the chopped tomato and
fry for about 10 minutes until
the liquid has reduced. Add the
spinach and continue to fry for
about two minutes until the
spinach starts to wilt
4 Lightly beat the eggs with salt
and pepper to taste and pour
over the vegetables in the frying
pan. Cook over a low heat until
the base of the omelette has set.
Cook the top under the grill
until it is set
5 Serve sprinkled with chopped
herbs and chives.

PREPARATION TIME:
5 minutes/COOKING TIME:
15 minutes

SPICY VEGETABLE AND TOFU OMELETTE (5)
CORE INGREDIENT
3 eggs
60 gm firm tofu, cut into
  small cubes

FRUIT/VEGETABLES
8–12 small shitake mushrooms
  or fresh baby mushrooms
1 tsp ginger
3–4 spring onions, chopped
2 cups spinach
1 cup bean sprouts
10–12 green beans, cut in half
2–3 cloves garlic

FROM THE CUPBOARD
1 T water
1 T mirin (optional)
2 T olive oil
1 T sesame oil
1 T soya sauce

HERBS AND SPICES
1 red chilli
2 tsp black pepper

1 If using dried shitake mushrooms pour boiling water over them and leave them to soak for about 20 minutes while preparing the rest of the omelette
2 Chop the garlic, ginger and chilli
3 Lightly beat together the eggs, water, mirin and black pepper
4 In a frying pan heat the olive and sesame oils over medium heat, add the garlic, ginger and chilli, mushrooms and beans and stir-fry for 2 to 3 minutes
5 Add the spring onions, tofu and soya sauce and fry until the sauce has almost evaporated (about 5 minutes)

6 Add the spinach and bean sprouts. Cover the pan and cook for about 1 minute until the spinach starts to wilt
7 Reduce the heat and pour over the egg mixture. Cook until the bottom of the omelette is set and then put the pan under the grill to finish off the top.

Serve with soya sauce and chilli sambal as accompaniments.

PREPARATION TIME: 2–3 minutes, plus 20 minutes soaking if using dried mushrooms/COOKING TIME: 10–12 minutes

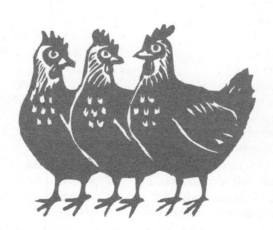

5.5 SOMETHING SAVOURY

Breakfast is often a neglected opportunity to be adventurous. Here is a selection of mouthwatering savoury Western and Asian breakfasts for you to try.

GRILLED MUSHROOMS ON TOAST (3)

CORE INGREDIENT
8 large field mushrooms, cleaned and stalks removed

FRUIT/VEGETABLES
2 cloves garlic

FROM THE CUPBOARD
3 T olive oil
4 slices wholemeal bread, toasted

HERBS AND SPICES
20 gm wide-leafed parsley
1/2 tsp black pepper
salt to taste

1 Combine the oil, garlic, parsley and pepper in a small food processor, add salt to taste and blend for about 30 seconds to one minute until the mixture has the consistency of a coarse purée
2 Brush the purée over the mushrooms and grill the mushrooms until they are cooked through. Do not turn the mushrooms over
3 Serve on toasted wholemeal bread.

PREPARATION TIME:
3–4 minutes/COOKING TIME:
3–4 minutes

VARIATIONS:
● *Chop the mushrooms into thick slices and stir-fry in the olive oil mixture and serve with toast or plain boiled rice or grilled polenta (page 133–4)*
● *Serve on wholemeal toast spread with tomato paste*
● *Spread the paste directly on the bread and grill the mushrooms (you may want to reduce the garlic).*

INDONESIAN MUNG BEAN SOUP (3) WITH CHICKEN (6)

CORE INGREDIENT
2 cooked chicken breasts (optional)

FRUIT/VEGETABLES
120 gm fresh mung beans
100 gm bean sprouts
4 spring onions, chopped
1 small onion, chopped
4 cloves garlic, chopped
1/2 T fresh ginger
1 T lemon juice

FROM THE CUPBOARD
1 litre chicken or vegetable
  stock
2 T olive oil

HERBS AND SPICES
1 tsp cumin
1 T coriander
1/2 tsp turmeric
1 tsp salt
1 tsp black pepper
1 red chilli (or to taste)

1 Fry the onion gently in a
saucepan until it turns
translucent, add the garlic,
ginger and chilli and continue
stir-frying on medium heat for
another minute. Add all the
spices and fry for another 1 to
2 minutes
2 Slowly add the stock to the
spice mix stirring to mix
thoroughly and simmer for
about 10 minutes
3 Divide the mung beans, bean
sprouts, chopped spring onion
and shredded cooked chicken
between 4 soup bowls
4 Pour the soup over the
chicken and vegetables. Garnish
with chopped coriander.

Serve with cooked rice in
separate bowls. Eat it the
Eastern way by picking up a
spoonful and dunking it in the
soup to moisten it.

PREPARATION TIME:
5 minutes/COOKING TIME:
15 minutes

SIMPLE MISO SOUP (1)

Miso is made by fermenting
soya, barley or other cereals.
It is the basis of a delicate soup
that is the mainstay of the
traditional, light breakfast of
Japan. It is very quick and easy
to make and very delicious. It is
especially good for those being
treated for, or recovering from,
cancer. It is also very good for
those on a slimming diet!

CORE INGREDIENT
100 gm bean curd, cut into cubes

FRUIT/VEGETABLES
2–3 spring onions, chopped
2 medium mushrooms, sliced

FROM THE CUPBOARD
1 litre chicken or vegetable
  stock
4 T Miso paste (reddish brown)

1 Bring the stock to a slow
simmer, add the bean curd and
continue to simmer for 2 to 3
minutes
2 Remove the pan from the
heat, add the miso and stir well
3 Serve with the spring onion
and mushrooms.

PREPARATION TIME:
2–3 minutes/COOKING TIME:
5–6 minutes

VARIATION:
● *Use traditional Japanese dashi as the stock.*

DASHI (0)
CORE INGREDIENT
5 cm kombu (Japanese
  seaweed)

FROM THE CUPBOARD
3 T dried bonito flakes
4–6 cups water

1 Wash the kombu
2 Add the water and kombu to a saucepan, bring to the boil and simmer for 2 to 3 minutes, then remove the kombu. (Some cooks recommend that the kombu be removed as soon as the water boils)
3 Add the bonito flakes, bring the water back to the boil, then remove immediately from the heat
4 Strain the soup.

PREPARATION TIME:
1 minute/COOKING TIME:
5 minutes

POTATO, AVOCADO AND BACON STACKS (7) – OR WITHOUT THE BACON (2)
This is our delicious substitute for eggs Benedict. Another great weekend breakfast/brunch. Just leave out the bacon if you have active cancer.

CORE INGREDIENT
4–8 slices unsmoked back bacon (optional)

FRUIT/VEGETABLES
2–3 large cooked potatoes,
  thickly sliced
2 avocados, peeled and sliced
1 T lemon juice
2 cloves garlic
1/2 small red onion, peeled and
  coarsely chopped
2 large tomatoes, thickly sliced

FROM THE CUPBOARD
2 T olive oil
8–12 sundried or sunblush
  tomatoes
1 T dairy-free basil pesto

HERBS AND SPICES
salt and pepper to taste
2 T fresh basil or parsley,
  chopped
1 tsp cayenne pepper (optional)

1 Add the avocado, onion, garlic, lemon juice, olive oil and cayenne pepper to a food processor and blend until it has the consistency of a smooth paste. Season to taste

2 Grill the bacon slices until crispy and lightly grill the tomato slices

3 At the same time sauté the potato slices in olive oil until they become crisp

4 Serve as a sandwich with a potato slice spread thickly with the avocado mixture, followed by the tomato and bacon slices and another slice of potato. Garnish with a few sundried or sunblush tomatoes, a sprinkle of basil or parsley pesto and some finely chopped basil or parsley leaves.

PREPARATION TIME:
10 minutes/COOKING TIME:
10 minutes

SHORT CUT: If you don't have time to make the avocado mix, just mash the avocado with a little lemon juice and serve on top of the potato slices

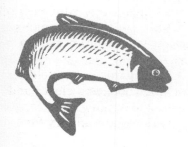

PESTO IS VERY EASY TO MAKE BY BLENDING 2 TO 3 GARLIC CLOVES, 2 CUPS OF FRESH BASIL, CORIANDER OR PARSLEY LEAVES, 1/2 CUP OF PINE NUTS AND 1/4 TO 1/2 CUP OF OLIVE OIL TOGETHER IN A FOOD PROCESSOR. IT KEEPS WELL IN THE FRIDGE FOR SEVERAL DAYS. WE HAVE FOUND A COMMERCIAL PESTO THAT CONTAINS NO DAIRY IN THE JEWISH SECTION OF THE SUPERMARKET, SO THIS CAN SUBSTITUTE FOR FRESHLY MADE PESTO IF YOU DO NOT HAVE THE TIME OR THE INGREDIENTS TO HAND.

OLD-FASHIONED KEDGEREE (6)

CORE INGREDIENT
250 gm smoked haddock or cod (optional)
2 eggs, hard boiled

FRUIT/VEGETABLES
1 small onion, chopped
3–4 garlic cloves, chopped
1 cup frozen peas
1 cup frozen corn
1 green or red pepper, chopped

FROM THE CUPBOARD

1 cup basmati rice or 2 1/2 cups
  cooked rice
4 T olive oil

HERBS AND SPICES

1 tsp turmeric
2 T chopped parsley

1 Cook 1 cup of rice in 2 cups
water (page 124) and add the
turmeric or sauté cooked rice in
olive oil with the turmeric until
it is warmed through
2 Poach or steam the fish until
it flakes easily (about 5 minutes)
3 At the same time heat the
olive oil, add the chopped onion
and cook until it is translucent.
Add the garlic, peas, corn and red
pepper and gently heat through
4 Put the flaked fish into a bowl.
Add the rice, chopped eggs,
onion and vegetables with any
oil that is left in the frying pan.
Mix together, season to taste,
and garnish with chopped
parsley.

PREPARATION TIME:
2–3 minutes/COOKING TIME:
15 minutes if cooking rice,
otherwise 5–6 minutes

RICE WITH LENTILS – INDIAN-STYLE KEDGEREE (3)

CORE INGREDIENT

1 cup of long grain rice

FRUIT/VEGETABLES

2–3 cloves garlic, chopped
1 T ginger, chopped
2 medium onions, chopped

FROM THE CUPBOARD

1/2 cup yellow lentils
4 T olive or sunflower oil
3 cups water
1/2 cup pine nuts or almonds

HERBS AND SPICES

1 red or green chilli, chopped
1 cinnamon stick
4–6 cloves
1/2 tsp turmeric
1/2 tsp cayenne pepper
salt to taste

1 Toast the pine nuts or
almonds either in the oven or in
a small frying pan
2 Wash and drain the rice and
lentils
3 Heat the olive or sunflower oil
in a saucepan, add the onions
and stir-fry until they start to
turn brown
4 Add the garlic, ginger, chilli,
cinnamon stick and cloves and
fry for 2 to 3 minutes
5 Add the lentils and fry for

about 2 minutes stirring to coat them in the oil and to stop them sticking to the pan

6 Add the water and turmeric and season to taste. Cover the pan and leave the lentils to simmer for about 15 minutes, then add the rice and continue to simmer until the water has been absorbed and the rice and lentils are tender. If the pan goes dry before the rice and lentils are cooked just add a little more water

7 Garnish with the chopped coriander and toasted nuts.

PREPARATION TIME:
5 minutes/COOKING TIME:
30–40 minutes

SIMPLE SAVOURY BREAKFAST SUGGESTIONS

- Grilled tomato on wholemeal toast (3)
- Hummus on toast (3)
- Home-made baked beans (page 141–2) (4)
- Vietnamese vegetable noodle soup (page 80–1) (3)

5.6 BREADS AND SPREADS

Dairy-free toast and jam, or other spreads such as organic peanut butter, are fine for breakfast, although check the salt, refined sugar and preservative content before buying. Rice or oatcakes can be substituted for wheat-grained breads if you prefer to follow a gluten-free diet.

Making bread and jam sounds daunting and time consuming for busy people, but it is worth it in the end! Here are some simple recipes for breads and jams you might want to try. You can make the bread when you have time and store it in the freezer for up to a week.

You can buy good organic jams and marmalades, including ones with no added sugar. But, here are a couple to get you started if you would like to make your own. Once made, the jam will keep for months.

STRAWBERRY PRESERVE (3)
CORE INGREDIENT
1 kg strawberries

FRUIT/VEGETABLES
juice of 4 lemons

FROM THE CUPBOARD
2 cups of raw cane sugar
2 tsp balsamic vinegar

1 Simmer hulled strawberries with the lemon juice in a large saucepan for about 25 minutes. Add the sugar and vinegar and stir until the sugar dissolves
2 Increase the heat and boil the jam rapidly for about 15 minutes stirring frequently to avoid it sticking to the pan and burning
3 Test the jam by putting a teaspoonful on a cold saucer to see if it sets. If it does not set, add a little more sugar and boil rapidly for another 5 minutes. If all else fails, reserve and use it as a sauce over soya 'ice cream', or our delicious home-made sorbets, or with pancakes
4 Spoon it into sterilised jars – the quantities here make about 5 jars.

PREPARATION TIME: 5 minutes/COOKING TIME: 45 minutes

APRICOT PRESERVE (3)
CORE INGREDIENT
1 kg apricots

FRUIT/VEGETABLES
juice of 2 lemons

FROM THE CUPBOARD
1 1/4 –1 1/2 cups of raw cane sugar
3 cups water

1 Cut the apricots in half, remove the stones, crack them open and remove the kernel
2 Blanch the kernels in hot water for about 5 minutes and then use strong nutcrackers to split them open. Geologists like us use our hammers! Wrap them in a piece of cheesecloth and twist into a little bag and seal with a rubber band
3 Quarter the apricots, add them to a large saucepan with the water, lemon juice and bag of kernels and simmer until they turn into a gel – about 1 1/2 hours
4 Add the sugar, take out the bag of kernels and fast boil the apricot gel for 15 minutes, stirring to ensure it doesn't burn
5 Ladle into sterilised jam jars and seal.

PREPARATION TIME: 10 minutes/COOKING TIME: 1 3/4 hours

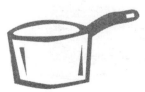

*TO STERILISE JAM JARS –
WASH THEM IN HOT
WATER AND DRY THEM
IN THE OVEN; EVEN
IF YOU USE THE
DISHWASHER THEY
SHOULD STILL BE
FINISHED OFF
IN THE OVEN.*

This quantity makes about
800 gm jam, or about 4 to 5 jars
depending on their size. The
jam does not set solid but can be
spread on bread and is delicious
without being too sweet.

ORANGE LEMON AND LIME MARMALADE WITH WHISKY (3)

This should be made with
unwaxed fruit.

CORE INGREDIENT
1 thin-skinned orange

FRUIT/VEGETABLES
2 small thin-skinned lemons
1 lime
1 medium carrot

FROM THE CUPBOARD
1 cup of raw cane sugar
1 cup of soft brown cane sugar
3 cups of water
3 T whisky (optional)

1 Wash and coarsely chop the
fruit and peel the carrot
2 Put the fruit and carrot into a
food processor with one cup of
water and process it until it is
all chopped finely
3 Add the fruit mixture to a
large saucepan, add the rest of
the water and the sugar, and
bring to the boil, then reduce
the heat and simmer for 30
minutes stirring occasionally
4 Turn up the heat and boil
rapidly for another 15–20
minutes watching carefully to
ensure it does not burn. You
should not have any problem
getting this to gel – our first
attempt was rock solid!
5 When the fruit has finished
boiling add the whisky, stir, ladle
into the sterilised jars and seal.

PREPARATION TIME:
15 minutes/COOKING TIME:
45–50 mins

WHISKY AND GINGER MARMALADE (3)

This is a much more complicated recipe and takes more time but it is truly degenerate!

CORE INGREDIENT
1 kg Seville oranges

FRUIT/VEGETABLES
juice of 1 lemon

FROM THE CUPBOARD
3 T whisky
3 cups of raw cane sugar
3 cups of water

HERBS AND SPICES
2 T preserved ginger, coarsely chopped

1 Wash and dry the oranges. Peel and coarsely chop the flesh and cut the peel into chunky slices and add to the orange pieces
2 Place the oranges and peel in a thick-bottomed, non-stick saucepan, add the lemon juice and sufficient water to cover the fruit mix by about 5 cm
3 Bring to the boil and simmer gently for 2 hours, stirring occasionally
4 Add the sugar, stirring gently until it is all dissolved
5 Simmer for another 30 minutes before adding the chopped ginger and continue to simmer for another 30 minutes
6 Remove from the heat, add the whisky and leave to cool for 15 minutes
7 Ladle into warm sterilised jars and seal.

PREPARATION TIME:
15–20 minutes/COOKING TIME: 3 hours

CHRIS'S BEER BREAD (3)

Chris Williams contributed this very quick and simple bread that requires no rising agent (no yeast). Its character comes from the beer – any kind, just experiment! It is great when spread with dairy-free pesto paste and/or humus. It also makes terrific (and very rich) French toast.

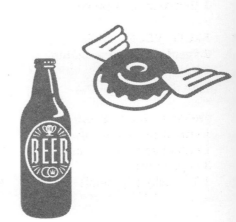

CORE INGREDIENT
500 gm self-raising wholemeal
 flour

FROM THE CUPBOARD
2 tsp olive oil
1 tsp cream of tartar (optional)
330 ml beer, preferably lager

HERBS AND SPICES
2 tsp salt

1 Mix flour, salt and cream of
tartar in a large bowl
2 Slowly add the olive oil and
rub it into the dry mix with
your fingertips
3 Make a well in the flour
mixture and pour the beer into
it and mix well, until the dough
is stiff, but not flaky dry
4 Knead the dough by hand for
a few minutes until the dough
is springy and elastic
5 Place the dough on a
worktop and form it into
the shape of a cylinder
6 Preheat the oven to 220°C.
Put the dough on a lightly oiled
baking tray and bake for about
35 to 40 minutes. Remove from
the oven, place on a rack and
cool for at least 15 minutes.

PREPARATION TIME:
15 minutes/COOKING TIME:
35–40 minutes, plus 15 minutes
to stand

OLIVE BREAD (3)

This is a traditional bread
that requires yeast and takes
time to rise. However, you will
be rewarded by a beautifully
flavoured bread that goes well
with any savoury spread. If you
want a classical breakfast
bread that goes well with jam or
marmalade just leave out
the olives and rosemary.

CORE INGREDIENT
600 gm strong flour

FROM THE CUPBOARD
4 T olive oil
100 gm de-stoned, black olives,
 coarsely chopped
1 T instant dried, active yeast
1 tsp sugar
300 ml warm water

HERBS AND SPICES
2 tsp salt
2 T finely chopped fresh
 rosemary

1 Dissolve the yeast, with the sugar, in about half of the warm water, or according to the instructions on the packet

2 Mix the flour, olives, salt and rosemary in a large bowl

3 Add the olive oil and the dissolved yeast to the rest of the warm water, pour into a well in the flour mixture, and mix well

4 Knead the dough, either by hand for 15 minutes, or with a dough hook, or in a bread maker until the dough is springy and elastic

5 If hand kneading place the dough in a lightly oiled bowl, cover with a clean tea towel and leave in a draught-free place to double in size (about 45 minutes)

6 If using a bread maker use the dough setting and leave for 1 hour and 45 minutes

7 Put the kneaded dough gently on your workbench, roll into the shape of a cylinder with oiled hands, place on a floured tea towel and allow to rise for another 30 minutes

8 Preheat the oven to 220°C with a baking tray in it. Roll the dough on to the hot baking tray, sprinkle with seasalt, and bake for 25 to 30 minutes.

PREPARATION TIME:
20 minutes, plus 75 minutes for rising / COOKING TIME: 25–30 minutes

VARIATIONS:
● *Use chopped sundried tomatoes and basil, instead of olives and rosemary.*
● *Use raisins and chopped walnuts, instead of olives and rosemary.*

6 Meals on the run

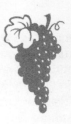

QUICK AND EASY, NUTRITIOUS, LIGHT AND SNACK MEALS

- Delightful soups based on fresh vegetables
- Lots of different crunchy salad vegetables and fruit
- Salad dressings based on high-quality vegetable oils and vinegars
- Cheese replaced with yummy home-made dips and spreads
- Dairy-free breads, oat and rice cakes
- Freshly shelled nuts and dried fruit
- Soya-based fruit yoghurt and drinks
- Herbal teas

MAKE AND TAKE YOUR OWN LUNCH RATHER THAN BUY

Most people's busy lifestyles mean that they and their families frequently eat ready-made snacks, especially at lunchtime. Relying on plastic-wrapped sandwiches, indifferent salads, or reheated, overcooked, baked potatoes is not good for anyone's health. Try to think ahead and work with the family to make meals to take with you. Make this a family event where you discuss and share ideas and communicate the idea that good food is central to good living.

Here are some great ideas for delicious light meals to stop you reaching for those two old dairy staples, cheese and yoghurt.

6.1 SUPER SOUPS

Many of these soups are nutritious meals in themselves, and they also make delicious starters for main meals and dinner parties. We have used coconut milk, potatoes or cauliflower to thicken them so you should not miss your cream, milk or cornflour. If, however, there are some soups you would prefer as 'cream of', then simply add a spoonful of soya cream to serve.

BARLEY AND LENTIL SOUP (3)

Peter Simpson, Jane's husband, made this soup for her during her chemotherapy treatment. She found it palatable and digestible even when she felt unable to eat most other things. It is a mild soup with a full range of protein and lots of vitamins and minerals.

This soup can be made either as a thick vegetable soup or a thinner broth by adjusting the quantities of ingredients.

CORE INGREDIENT
1/2 cup red lentils

FRUIT/VEGETABLES
2 onions, chopped
4 carrots, chopped
A thick slice of turnip, chopped
2 small potatoes, chopped

FROM THE CUPBOARD
2 T olive oil
1/3 cup pearl barley
1 1/2 L vegetable stock

HERBS AND SPICES
2 T chopped parsley
2 T chopped chives

1 Heat the oil, add all the vegetables and sauté for 3 to 4 minutes until the onions are soft and translucent
2 Add the stock, lentils and barley and simmer for 20 minutes until the lentils and barley are soft
3 Serve sprinkled with the parsley and chives.

It tastes even better if left overnight, add the parsley and chives just before serving.

PREPARATION TIME:
5–6 minutes/COOKING TIME:
25 minutes

BEAN SOUP (3)

CORE INGREDIENT
1 can chickpeas

FRUIT/VEGETABLES
1 onion
3–4 cloves of garlic, chopped

FROM THE CUPBOARD
2 T olive oil
1 can red kidney beans
1 can cannellini beans
1/2 cup fresh or frozen
  broad beans
1/2 cup olive oil
1/2 cup tomato paste
1 L vegetable stock

HERBS AND SPICES
1 T ground cumin
1 T ground coriander
1/2 tsp cayenne pepper

1/2 cup fresh chopped coriander
salt and pepper to taste

1 Heat the oil in a saucepan and
sauté the onion for 2 to 3
minutes
2 Add the garlic, tomato paste,
cumin, coriander and chilli and
continue to sauté for another
minute
3 Add the stock, bring to the
boil, turn down the heat and
simmer for 10 minutes
4 Add the chickpeas and beans
and continue to simmer for
another 10 to 15 minutes until
the beans are soft
5 Season to taste and serve
garnished with chopped
coriander.

PREPARATION TIME:
2–3 minutes/COOKING TIME:
25–30 minutes

BROCCOLI AND CAULIFLOWER SOUP (3)
CORE INGREDIENT
500 gm mixed broccoli and
cauliflower, cut into florets

FRUIT/VEGETABLES
2 medium onions, chopped
8–10 cloves garlic, minced

FROM THE CUPBOARD
2 T olive oil
1 L chicken or vegetable stock

HERBS AND SPICES
salt and black pepper to taste
2 T chopped chives
2 T chopped parsley

1 Heat the oil and fry the onion
for 2 to 3 minutes, then add the
garlic, cauliflower and broccoli
and continue to fry for another
1 to 2 minutes stirring to coat
the vegetables with the oil
2 Add the stock, season to taste
and simmer for about 10
minutes or until the vegetables
are tender
3 Eat it as it is or puréed in a
food processor
4 Serve sprinkled with fresh
chopped chives and parsley.

PREPARATION TIME:
6–8 minutes/COOKING TIME:
15–20 minutes

PEEL AND SLICE BROCCOLI STALKS AND USE THEM IN SOUPS OR ANY VEGETABLE CASSEROLE DISH.

CANNELLINI BEAN AND LENTIL SOUP (3)
CORE INGREDIENT
1 can cannellini beans, drained
and rinsed

FRUIT/VEGETABLES
1 large onion, chopped

3–4 cloves garlic, minced
5 fresh ripe tomatoes, chopped
1 large stalk celery, sliced
1 medium zucchini, sliced
1 green pepper, sliced

FROM THE CUPBOARD
2 T olive oil
2 T tomato paste
1/2 cup green 'puy' lentils
1 L chicken or vegetable stock
125 gm egg noodles

HERBS AND SPICES
salt and pepper
1 tsp cayenne pepper
2 T chopped coriander or
parsley

1 Heat the oil and sauté the
onion for 2 to 3 minutes before
adding the garlic and sautéing
for another minute
2 Add the celery, tomatoes,
zucchini, green pepper, tomato
paste and cayenne pepper and
sauté for 2 to 3 minutes
3 Pour in the stock and lentils
and simmer for about 20
minutes or until the lentils
are soft
4 Add the egg noodles and
cannellini beans, season to taste
and simmer for 4 to 5 minutes
until the egg noodles are
cooked
5 Serve garnished with chopped
coriander or parsley.

PREPARATION TIME:
5–10 minutes/COOKING TIME:
30 minutes

CARROT AND ORANGE SOUP (3)
CORE INGREDIENT
500 gm carrots, peeled and
coarsely chopped

FRUIT/VEGETABLES
1 onion, finely chopped
1 leek, finely chopped
juice of 2 oranges
2–3 cloves garlic, minced

FROM THE CUPBOARD
2 T olive oil
1 1/2 L chicken or vegetable stock
1 T sherry vinegar

HERBS AND SPICES
salt and pepper
2 T chopped chives
2 T chopped parsley

1 Heat the oil in a saucepan,
add the garlic and vegetables
and sauté gently for about five
minutes
2 Add the stock, vinegar and
orange juice and simmer until
the carrot is very soft
3 Purée the soup and season to
taste
4 Serve sprinkled with fresh
chives and parsley.

PREPARATION TIME:
5 minutes/COOKING TIME:
15–20 minutes

VARIATION:
● *This soup is also
delicious served cold.*

COCONUT AND
CHICKEN SOUP (6)
CORE INGREDIENT
2 chicken breasts, cubed
  (optional)

FRUIT/VEGETABLES
3–4 cloves garlic
2 T fresh ginger or Thai ginger
  (galangal – now available in
  some good Chinese grocery
  shops)
2 shallots, peeled
8 baby corn, halved
4 stalks asparagus, cut into 3 cm
  lengths
8 baby mushrooms, halved
1/2 cup bean sprouts
3 T lime or lemon juice
1 small red pepper, sliced
2 spring onions, chopped

FROM THE CUPBOARD
1 T peanut or sunflower oil
2 cups coconut milk
1 L vegetable or chicken stock
1 T fish sauce

HERBS AND SPICES
2 stalks lemon grass

2 green chillies
1 tsp salt
3–4 lime leaves
black pepper
fresh coriander including the
  roots if possible

1 Chop the garlic, ginger,
shallots, chilli, coriander roots,
black pepper and olive oil in a
blender or food processor until
it forms a smooth paste. Add a
little of the coconut milk if
necessary
2 Add the paste, lemon grass
and lime leaves to a saucepan
and stir-fry briefly for 2 to 3
minutes
3 Add the corn, asparagus, red
pepper and chicken and stir-fry
until the chicken is seared
4 Slowly add the coconut milk
and simmer uncovered until the
chicken is cooked
5 Add the bean sprouts, spring
onions, fish sauce and lime juice
and cook for another minute
6 Garnish with chopped
coriander and serve with
steamed rice.

PREPARATION TIME: 10 mins
COOKING TIME: 20 mins

VARIATION:
● *Make the soup with chicken or
vegetable stock alone rather than
adding coconut milk*

IT IS IMPORTANT NOT TO BOIL COCONUT MILK, JUST SIMMER IT GENTLY AND ALWAYS COOK IT UNCOVERED, OR IT WILL SEPARATE.

COCONUT AND PRAWN SOUP (6)

CORE INGREDIENT
16–20 green prawns

FRUIT/VEGETABLES
1 small onion, roughly chopped
1 fennel bulb, sliced
1 T garlic, chopped
1 T ginger, minced
2 T lemon juice
1 red pepper, sliced
2 cups of spinach
1/2 can bamboo shoots

FROM THE CUPBOARD
2 T olive oil
1 L chicken stock
2 cups coconut milk

HERBS AND SPICES
2 T paprika
1 red chilli
1 tsp ground coriander
1/2 tsp coarse ground black pepper
1/4 tsp ground fenugreek (optional)
1/2 tsp salt

1 Heat the oil and fry the onion for 3 to 4 minutes, add the fennel, garlic, ginger and other spices and continue to fry for another 1 to 2 minutes

2 Add the chicken stock, bring to a boil, cover and simmer for about 15 minutes, then remove from the heat and purée

3 Return to the heat, add the prawns, bamboo shoots and red pepper and simmer for 2 to 3 minutes

4 Add the coconut milk and bring to a simmer then add the spinach and beansprouts and cook until the spinach is just wilted

5 Stir in the lemon juice and serve sprinkled with chopped coriander.

PREPARATION TIME:
6–7 minutes/COOKING TIME:
25–30 minutes

CORN SOUP (3)

CORE INGREDIENT
2 cups of corn kernels

FRUIT/VEGETABLES
2–3 cloves garlic, minced
1 large onion, chopped

FROM THE CUPBOARD
2 T olive oil
1 L vegetable or chicken stock

HERBS AND SPICES
salt and pepper to taste
1–2 T chopped parsley
1 T cumin powder

1 Heat the oil and sauté the onion for 2 to 3 minutes, then add the garlic and stir-fry for another minute
2 Add the stock, bring to the boil and simmer for 10 minutes
3 Add the corn and simmer for another 10 minutes until the corn is tender
4 Purée, season to taste, and serve with chopped parsley and swirl in a little cumin powder.

PREPARATION TIME:
2–3 minutes/COOKING TIME:
25 minutes

GAZPACHO SOUP (4)
Because this lovely summer soup consists entirely of fresh vegetables, its flavour depends on using the very best ingredients.
CORE INGREDIENT
4–5 medium tomatoes

FRUIT/VEGETABLES
2–3 cloves garlic
1 large red onion, peeled
1/2 cucumber, peeled
1 red pepper, seeded and
  coarsely chopped

FROM THE CUPBOARD
1 can tomato juice
2 T red wine vinegar
1/2 –1 cup water
3–4 T olive oil

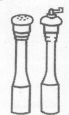

HERBS AND SPICES
salt and pepper

1 Put all the ingredients, except the water and salt and pepper, in a food processor and process until smooth
2 Add enough water to dilute to a 'soupy' consistency and season to taste
3 Chill before serving
4 Serve with ice cubes and bowls of chopped tomato, cucumber, green and red pepper and onion as garnishes.

PREPARATION TIME:
15 minutes

JAPANESE NOODLE SOUP WITH PRAWNS (6)
CORE INGREDIENT
3–4 medium prawns per person

FRUIT/VEGETABLES
2 spring onions, chopped
1 cup mushrooms, sliced

FROM THE CUPBOARD
1 L dashi (page 53) or chicken
  stock
1/2 cup mirin

¹/₂ cup Japanese soya sauce
125 gm fresh egg noodles

HERBS AND SPICES
2 T fresh coriander, chopped

1 Mix together the dashi or stock, mirin and soya sauce and simmer for 10 minutes
2 Add the noodles, prawns and mushrooms and continue to simmer for 3 to 4 minutes until the prawns turn pink
3 Add the spring onions and fresh coriander and serve.

PREPARATION TIME:
2–3 minutes/COOKING TIME:
15 minutes

MINTED PEA AND POTATO SOUP
CORE INGREDIENT
600 gm potato, diced

FRUIT/VEGETABLES
200 gm leek, finely sliced
500 gm frozen peas
3–4 garlic cloves, sliced

FROM THE CUPBOARD
2 T olive oil
1¹/₂ L chicken or vegetable stock

HERBS AND SPICES
salt and pepper
¹/₂ cup mint or parsley, chopped

1 Heat the oil and sauté the leeks, potato and garlic for about 4 to 5 minutes
2 Add the stock, season to taste and simmer until the potatoes are cooked (about 20 minutes)
3 Add the peas and heat through
4 Purée to a smooth consistency
5 Bring the soup back to a simmer and serve with chopped mint or parsley.

PREPARATION TIME:
5 minutes/COOKING TIME:
25–30 minutes

MIXED VEGETABLE SOUP (3)
As with all vegetable soups, this can be made with any vegetables, so use what you have left in the fridge.

CORE INGREDIENT
1 L chicken or vegetable stock

FRUIT/VEGETABLES
3–4 cloves garlic, chopped
1 small onion, finely chopped
¹/₂ tin bamboo shoots
100 gm baby corn, cut in half
1 zucchini, sliced
1 cup of broccoli florets

FROM THE CUPBOARD
1 T olive oil
2 T fish sauce

HERBS AND SPICES
1/2 cup Thai basil or coriander
  and/or chives, finely chopped

1 Heat the oil in a saucepan
and sauté the onion for 2 to 3
minutes, add the garlic and
continue to cook for another
minute
2 Add the stock and all the
other ingredients except the
Thai basil or coriander and
simmer for about 10 minutes
until the vegetables are just
cooked
3 Serve garnished with the Thai
basil or coriander and/or chives.

PREPARATION TIME:
4–5 minutes/COOKING TIME:
15 minutes

MUSHROOM SOUP (3)
CORE INGREDIENT
250 gm fresh shitake
  mushrooms, sliced
200 gm chestnut mushrooms,
  sliced

FRUIT/VEGETABLES
2 potatoes, cubed
3–4 cloves garlic, minced
1 T lemon juice

FROM THE CUPBOARD
2 T walnut oil
1 L vegetable stock
1 cup dry white wine (optional)

HERBS AND SPICES
salt and pepper to taste
2 T chopped parsley

1 Add the potatoes to a
saucepan with the stock and
wine and simmer until the
potatoes are cooked
2 Heat the oil in a pan and
sauté the garlic and mushrooms
for 2 to 3 minutes
3 Add the mushrooms to the
stock and purée until smooth
4 Stir in the lemon juice
5 Season to taste and serve
with chopped parsley.

PREPARATION TIME:
5 minutes/COOKING TIME:
20 minutes

NOODLE SOUP WITH MISO (3) AND CHICKEN (6)
CORE INGREDIENT
2 chicken breasts, sliced
  (optional)

FRUIT/VEGETABLES
100 gm kai lan, cut into 3 pieces
4 spring onions, chopped
100 gm bean sprouts

FROM THE CUPBOARD
2 tsp fish sauce
2 T soya sauce
1 1/2 L water
200 gm fresh egg noodles
4 T miso paste

1 Bring the fish sauce, soya and water to the boil in a saucepan
2 Turn down the heat before adding the sliced chicken pieces and simmer for 3 to 4 minutes until the chicken is just cooked
3 Add the kai lan and egg noodles and cook for a further 2 to 3 minutes until the noodles are just tender
4 Add the bean sprouts and spring onions, stir and heat through for one minute
5 Turn off the heat, add the miso, and stir until it is thoroughly mixed
6 Serve garnished with chopped coriander.

PREPARATION TIME:
3–4 minutes/COOKING TIME:
10 minutes

ONION AND GARLIC SOUP (3)
CORE INGREDIENT
6 medium brown onions, sliced

FRUIT/VEGETABLES
5–6 cloves garlic, minced

FROM THE CUPBOARD
2–3 T olive oil
1 L vegetable, or chicken stock
1 cup red wine (optional)

HERBS AND SPICES
salt and pepper

2 T chopped chives

1 Heat the olive oil, add the onions and fry over a low heat for about 15 minutes until the onions turn golden brown, then add the garlic and continue frying for 1 to 2 minutes
2 Add the stock and red wine, season to taste, cover and simmer for about 20 minutes
3 Serve garnished with chopped chives.

PREPARATION TIME:
10 minutes/COOKING TIME:
35–40 minutes

ONION AND POTATO SOUP (3)
CORE INGREDIENT
2 large onions, coarsely
    chopped

FRUIT/VEGETABLES
4–6 cloves garlic, minced
3 large potatoes, coarsely
    chopped

FROM THE CUPBOARD
2 T olive oil
1 L vegetable stock

HERBS AND SPICES
salt and pepper to taste
2 T chopped parsley or
    coriander

1 Heat the oil and add the onions, potatoes and garlic and sauté for about 5 minutes
2 Add the vegetable stock and salt and pepper to taste and simmer for about 20 minutes until the potatoes are very soft
3 Purée and serve garnished with chopped parsley or coriander.

PREPARATION TIME:
5–6 minutes/COOKING TIME:
25–30 minutes

VARIATIONS:
● *Add 1 large, coarsely chopped, fennel bulb.*
● *For a milder taste use leeks instead of onions and less garlic.*

SOUPS CAN BE PURÉED EITHER WITH A HAND-HELD BLENDER IN THE SAUCEPAN IN WHICH THEY HAVE BEEN COOKED, OR IN A FOOD PROCESSOR

PUMPKIN AND CORIANDER SOUP (3)
CORE INGREDIENT
1/2 pumpkin, peeled and cut into cubes

FRUIT/VEGETABLES
1 carrot, sliced
2 stick celery, sliced

1 leek, sliced
1 onion, chopped
4–5 cloves garlic, minced

FROM THE CUPBOARD
2 T olive oil
1 L chicken stock

HERBS AND SPICES
1 tsp ground cumin
1 tsp ground coriander
2 T fresh coriander
salt and pepper to taste

1 Heat the olive oil in a large saucepan, add the onion, pumpkin, leek and carrot and stir-fry for about 3 to 4 minutes
2 Add the garlic and ground spices and continue frying for another 1 to 2 minutes
3 Add the stock, bring to the boil and simmer for about 30 minutes
4 Purée to a smooth consistency
5 Season to taste and serve with chopped fresh coriander.

PREPARATION TIME:
10 minutes/COOKING TIME:
35 minutes

RED PEPPER SOUP (3)
CORE INGREDIENT
4 red peppers, seeded and chopped

FRUIT/VEGETABLES
1 onion, chopped
2 garlic cloves, minced

FROM THE CUPBOARD
3 T olive oil
1 L chicken stock

HERBS AND SPICES
1 red chilli, chopped
2 bay leaves
1 T chopped chives
salt and pepper to taste

1 Heat the oil and sauté the onions for 2 to 3 minutes, add the garlic, chilli and red pepper and continue cooking for another 1 to 2 minutes
2 Add the stock and bay leaves, season to taste and simmer for about 15–20 minutes
3 Remove the bay leaves and blend to a smooth purée
4 Serve garnished with chopped chives.

PREPARATION TIME: 5–6 mins
COOKING TIME: 20–25 mins

SIMPLE MULLIGATAWNY SOUP (3)
This is a delicious soup based on a traditional Indian recipe.

CORE INGREDIENT
1 cup green lentils, rinsed and drained

FRUIT/VEGETABLES
2 medium onions, peeled and chopped
3–4 cloves garlic, chopped
1 T fresh ginger, chopped

FROM THE CUPBOARD
3 T olive oil
1 cup coconut milk
1½ L chicken or vegetable stock
4 T cooked rice (optional)

HERBS AND SPICES
1 tsp cayenne pepper
1 tsp ground turmeric
1 tsp ground coriander
1 tsp ground cumin
2 bay leaves
2 T tamarind liquid
1 T garam masala
2 T fresh coriander

1 Soak 1 teaspoon of tamarind pulp in 2 tablespoons of boiling water for about 20 minutes, squeeze the pulp, strain and reserve the liquid
2 Heat the olive oil in a saucepan and fry the onion for about 3 to 4 minutes until it turns golden brown
3 Add the garlic, bay leaves, cayenne pepper, ground coriander, cumin and turmeric, and fry for 1 to 2 minutes, stirring to ensure the spices do not stick to the pan
4 Slowly add the coconut milk

and simmer for 2 minutes

5 Add the stock and rinsed, drained lentils, bring to the boil, cover and simmer for 30 minutes

6 Purée in a blender until smooth; add the reserved tamarind liquid, cooked rice and lemon juice, and bring back to the boil

7 Serve, sprinkled with garam masala and coriander leaves.

PREPARATION TIME: 5–6 minutes/COOKING TIME: 40–45 minutes

SPINACH (3) AND COD SOUP (6)

CORE INGREDIENT
125 gm cod or similar firm fish cut into cubes

FRUIT/VEGETABLES
4–6 cloves garlic, minced
1 T fresh ginger, minced
1/2 onion, chopped
juice of half a lemon
6–8 oyster mushrooms, cut into pieces
6–8 baby corn, halved
2 cups baby spinach leaves
1/2 red pepper, sliced

FROM THE CUPBOARD
2 T olive oil
1 L vegetable stock
60 gm rice vermicelli noodles

1 T fish sauce

HERBS AND SPICES
1 stick lemon grass, cut into 2 1/2 cm pieces
4–5 lime leaves
1 red chilli, chopped
2 T fresh coriander

1 Mix together the fish, fish sauce and ginger and leave to marinate for 10 to 15 minutes
2 Heat the olive oil, add the onion and stir-fry for 2 to 3 minutes then add the garlic, chilli, lemon grass, lime leaves and corn and continue to stir-fry for 2 to 3 minutes
3 Add the stock and bring to the boil
4 Turn down the heat, add the mushrooms and red pepper and simmer for 5 minutes
5 Add the fish and simmer for another 4 to 5 minutes, then add the spinach and noodles and cook for another 2 minutes
6 Season to taste and serve sprinkled with fresh chopped coriander.

PREPARATION TIME: 6–7 minutes/COOKING TIME: 20 minutes

VARIATION:
● *Add bean sprouts, or use chicken instead of cod*

SPINACH AND PRAWN SOUP (6)

CORE INGREDIENT

4–5 green king prawns per
  person

FRUIT/VEGETABLES

3–4 cloves garlic, minced
8 large shitake mushrooms
2 T lemon or lime juice
2 cups spinach
1/2 cup bamboo shoots
2 spring onions, chopped
8 snowpeas, halved
8 green beans, cut into 2 1/2 cm
  pieces

FROM THE CUPBOARD

1 tsp fish sauce
125 gm rice vermicelli
1 L chicken or vegetable stock

HERBS AND SPICES

1 red chilli, sliced
1 stalk lemon grass cut into 2 1/2
  cm pieces
2–3 lime leaves
2 T fresh coriander

1 If using dry shitake
mushrooms soak them in
boiling water for about 20
minutes, then drain and reserve
the liquid
2 Put the stock (and reserved
mushroom water) in a large
saucepan and add the garlic,
ginger, chilli, lemon grass and
lime leaves and simmer gently
for about 10 minutes
3 Add the beans, bamboo
shoots, and mushrooms and
continue to simmer for about 5
minutes
4 Add the prawns and simmer
until the prawns just turn pink,
about 2 to 3 minutes
5 Add the spinach, snowpeas,
spring onions and fish sauce
and simmer for another 1 to 2
minutes until the spinach is
wilted then stir in the lemon
juice
6 Pour boiling water over the
rice vermicelli and leave it to
stand for about 2 minutes, drain
and serve in individual soup
bowls
7 Ladle the soup over the
noodles, season to taste with salt
and pepper and garnish with
coriander.

PREPARATION TIME:
5–6 minutes/COOKING TIME:
20 minutes

VARIATION:
● *Omit the prawns and you have
a delicious Thai-style spinach soup.*

SWEET POTATO AND COCONUT SOUP (4)

CORE INGREDIENT

600 gm sweet potato, peeled and
cut into cubes

FRUIT/VEGETABLES
1 small onion, chopped
3–4 cloves garlic, minced
2 T lime or lemon juice
1 T ginger, chopped

FROM THE CUPBOARD
400 ml coconut milk
1 L vegetable or chicken stock
2 T olive oil

HERBS AND SPICES
1 red chilli, chopped
1 stalk lemon grass, cut into 2 1/2
  cm pieces
4 lime leaves
2 T fresh coriander, chopped

1 Heat the olive oil and stir-fry
the onion for 2 to 3 minutes
2 Add the garlic, ginger, chilli,
lemon grass and lime leaves and
continue to stir-fry for 1 to 2 mins
3 Pour in the coconut milk, stir
well and bring to a simmer
4 Add the sweet potato and
simmer for about 7 to 8 minutes
then add the stock and bring
back to a simmer
5 When the sweet potato is
tender remove the lime leaves
and lemon grass, blend the soup
then return to the heat
(alternatively blend the soup
and then strain)
6 Stir in the lime or lemon juice
and serve garnished with
coriander.

PREPARATION TIME:
6–7 minutes/COOKING TIME:
20–25 minutes

VARIATION:
● *Use pumpkin instead of*
sweet potato.

THAI-STYLE PRAWN SOUP (6)
This is the classic Thai soup
that really needs the lime
leaves and fresh lemon grass to
develop its fresh lemony and
hot flavour. We usually make it
with frozen green tiger prawns
from the freezer section in the
supermarket.

CORE INGREDIENT
16–20 medium green prawns

FRUIT/VEGETABLES
3 cloves garlic, minced
1 T fresh ginger, minced
2 T lime or lemon juice
4–6 spring onions, chopped
8–12 shitake, oyster or baby
  mushrooms, halved

FROM THE CUPBOARD
1 L chicken stock
2 tsp fish sauce

HERBS AND SPICES
2 red chillies, chopped
2 stalks lemon grass, cut into
  thick slices
2 T coriander roots, chopped

(optional)
1/2 tsp black pepper
3–4 fresh lime leaves
2 T fresh coriander or Thai
  basil leaves

1 Defrost and de-vein the prawns leaving the tail on
2 Bring the stock to a slow simmer, add the lemon grass, garlic, ginger, coriander root and lime leaves and simmer for about 15 mins
3 Strain the stock to remove the lemon grass and other seasonings, add the mushrooms and prawns and simmer until the prawns turn pink (about 3 minutes)
4 Add the spring onions, fish sauce, lime juice and finely chopped chilli, stir while heating through for about a minute
5 Serve garnished with fresh coriander or Thai basil.

PREPARATION TIME:
10 minutes/COOKING TIME:
20 minutes

TOMATO SOUP (3)
CORE INGREDIENT
5 large vine-ripened tomatoes,
  coarsely chopped

FRUIT/VEGETABLES
4–5 cloves garlic, finely chopped
2 small red onions, chopped

FROM THE CUPBOARD
2 T tomato paste
2 T olive oil
1 L vegetable stock

HERBS AND SPICES
1–2 red chillies, chopped
2 T parsley and basil, chopped
salt and pepper

1 Heat the olive oil and sauté the onion in a saucepan for 2 to 3 minutes
2 Add the garlic, tomato paste and chillies and continue to sauté for 1 to 2 minutes
3 Add the chopped tomatoes, season to taste and sauté for 2 to 3 minutes
4 Add the stock, bring to the boil, turn down the heat and gently simmer for 10 to 15 minutes
5 Purée and serve with chopped parsley and basil.

PREPARATION TIME:
3–4 minutes/COOKING TIME:
15–20 minutes

*CHOP ALL YOUR
PARSLEY IN ONE
SESSION AND STORE
IN A CONTAINER
IN THE FRIDGE.*

TRADITIONAL MINESTRONE (3)

The quantities in this recipe are only approximate. Use what you have – a little bit more, a little bit less does not matter. Every time you cook this soup it will taste slightly different but it is always good. It does take a long time to cook but after the preparation it looks after itself. It is delicious eaten immediately but even better after a day in the fridge so make plenty.

CORE INGREDIENT
4–5 vine-ripened tomatoes, chopped

FRUIT/VEGETABLES
1 medium onion, finely sliced
3–4 cloves garlic, minced
3 carrots, sliced
3 stalks celery, sliced
2 large potatoes, cubed
2 small/1 large zucchini, sliced
16–20 green beans, cut into 5 cm lengths
4–5 leaves Savoy cabbage, shredded

FROM THE CUPBOARD
4 T olive oil
1 1/2 L chicken or vegetable stock
1 can cannellini beans, drained and rinsed

HERBS AND SPICES
1 red chilli, chopped (optional)
1 tsp salt
1 tsp black pepper
2 bay leaves
3 T chopped parsley or basil

1 Heat the olive oil, add the onion and stir-fry for about 2 to 3 minutes, then add the garlic and chilli and continue to stir-fry for another 1 to 2 minutes
2 Add the carrots stirring to ensure they are well coated with oil
3 Next add the celery to the pot again stirring to cover in oil, and repeat in turn with the potatoes, zucchini, green beans and finally the sliced cabbage and stir well
4 Add the tomatoes, stock, salt, pepper and bay leaves. Lightly simmer for about 2 1/2 hours. (This can be interrupted at any time and the soup can be reheated later)
5 Add the cannellini beans about 15 minutes before serving, and warm through.
6 Garnish with chopped parsley and basil.

Serve with warm fresh bread.

PREPARATION TIME:
20 minutes/COOKING TIME:
2 1/2 hours

VEGETABLE NOODLE SOUP (3) WITH CHICKEN (6)

CORE INGREDIENT
2 chicken breasts, finely sliced

FRUIT/VEGETABLES
2–3 cloves garlic, chopped
1 T fresh ginger, chopped
6–8 fresh shitake or baby
  mushrooms, halved
1 cup bean sprouts
2 cups chopped Chinese greens
  or spinach
2–3 spring onions, chopped
1 T lemon juice

FROM THE CUPBOARD
1 T olive oil
1 L chicken or vegetable stock
60 gm rice or egg vermicelli

HERBS AND SPICES
1 tsp cumin powder
1/2 tsp turmeric
1/4 tsp shrimp paste
1 red chilli, chopped
2 T chopped coriander
salt to taste
1 tsp coarse black pepper

1 Heat the oil, add the garlic,
ginger, cumin powder, turmeric,
chilli and shrimp paste and stir-
fry for about 1 minute
2 Add the chicken and stir-fry
until it is seared before adding
the stock and simmering for
about 10 minutes (if using pre-

cooked chicken add it when you
add the noodles)
3 Add the noodles, mushrooms
and Chinese greens and simmer
for 2 to 3 minutes until the
greens are just cooked
4 Stir in the bean sprouts,
spring onions and lemon juice
and simmer for one more
minute
5 Serve garnished with
coriander.

PREPARATION TIME:
15 minutes/COOKING TIME:
15 minutes

VEGETABLES WITH BEAN CURD SOUP (3)

CORE INGREDIENT
1/2 packet bean curd cut
  into cubes

FRUIT/VEGETABLES
8–10 small shitake
  mushrooms or small
  fresh mushrooms
1 carrot, julienned
60 gm cauliflower, divided
  into florets
60 gm fresh baby corn, cut
  in half
1 T lemon juice
3–4 garlic cloves, minced
1 T fresh ginger, minced
3–4 spring onions,
  chopped

79

FROM THE CUPBOARD
1/2 T olive oil
2 T soya sauce
50 gm rice vermicelli
1 L vegetable stock

HERBS AND SPICES
2 T chopped fresh mint and/or
   coriander
1 red chilli, chopped
6 lime leaves
1 stick lemon grass, cut into 5
   cm pieces
salt and pepper to taste

1 If using dry shitake
mushrooms, put them in a bowl,
pour over boiling water and
leave them to soak for about 20
minutes then drain
2 Put the stock, garlic, ginger,
chilli, lime leaves and lemon
grass in a saucepan and simmer
for about 10 minutes
3 Strain the stock (optional),
then add the carrot, cauliflower,
corn and mushrooms and
simmer for five minutes
4 Add the noodles, bean curd
and soya sauce and simmer for
2 to 3 minutes until the noodles
are soft
5 Stir in the lemon juice, season
to taste.

Serve garnished with the fresh
mint or coriander.

PREPARATION TIME: 10–12 mins
COOKING TIME: 20 mins

VIETNAMESE-STYLE CHICKEN NOODLE SOUP (6)
CORE INGREDIENT
2 chicken breasts, thinly sliced

FRUIT/VEGETABLES
3–4 spring onions, sliced
1 T fresh ginger
1 T fresh lime juice
8–12 shitake or oyster
   mushrooms, halved
8–12 baby corn, halved
60 gm bean sprouts

FROM THE CUPBOARD
1 L chicken stock
100 gm egg noodles

HERBS AND SPICES
2 stalks lemon grass, finely
   chopped
4–5 lime leaves
1 red chilli, chopped
2 T chopped Thai basil or fresh
   coriander leaves

1 Steam the chicken breast until
it is cooked (about 15 minutes)
then slice thinly
2 Heat the stock with the
ginger, mushrooms, corn, lemon
grass, lime leaves and chilli and
simmer for about 10 minutes
3 Add the noodles and continue

to cook for 2 minutes
4 Just before serving add the spring onions, bean sprouts and lime juice, stir and cook for another minute
5 Divide the chicken between soup bowls, ladle the soup over it and garnish with fresh coriander or Thai basil.

PREPARATION TIME:
5 minutes/COOKING TIME:
15 minutes

6.2 SUMPTUOUS SALADS

With the fabulous fresh vegetables and fruit around these days, salads no longer have to mean a tasteless assemblage of limp lettuce leaf with chunks of cucumber and tomato and a dollop of bought salad cream. There is no excuse for today's salads not to be the beautifully coloured, textured and tasty 'salades' – in the French style. They can be prepared with a minimum of effort and because salads are packed with vitamins, antioxidants and anticancer chemicals they are so healthy. Simple, tasty salad dressings bring out the best in these delicious meals.

TRY TO HAVE AT LEAST ONE LARGE PLATE OF SALAD A DAY.

COLD SALADS

ASIAN-STYLE SALAD WITH PRAWNS (6)
CORE INGREDIENT
250 gm prawns

FRUIT/VEGETABLES
2 cloves garlic, crushed
1 T ginger, minced
1 red pepper, sliced
1 carrot, grated
8–12 baby corn, halved
4–6 spring onions, sliced
3–4 sticks celery, sliced
1 cup of bean sprouts

FROM THE CUPBOARD
3 T sesame oil
3 T soya sauce
2 T sesame seeds

HERBS AND SPICES
1 red chilli, chopped (optional)
2 T chopped herbs such as chives, basil and coriander

1 Peel and de-vein the prawns
2 Mix together the ginger, garlic, chilli, sesame oil and soya sauce, pour over the prawns and leave them to marinate for at least 30 minutes
3 Toast the sesame seeds in a

dry pan for 1 to 2 minutes until they just turn colour

4 Prepare all the salad vegetables, mix them together and divide between serving plates

5 Pour the prawns and marinade into a frying pan or wok and stir-fry for 2 to 3 minutes until the prawns just turn pink

6 Pour the prawns with their dressing over the salad and garnish with fresh herbs.

PREPARATION TIME: 10 minutes/COOKING TIME: 2–3 minutes

GREEN PRAWNS ARE OFTEN SOLD IN THEIR SHELLS. TO DE-VEIN, REMOVE THE SHELL FROM THE LEGS, LEAVING THE TAIL ON. YOU CAN EITHER GRAB THE BLACK VEIN THAT IS VISIBLE AT THE HEAD END OF THE PRAWN AND PEEL BACK, OR, IF YOU WANT THE TAILS OFF AND ARE REALLY CLEVER, GENTLY SQUEEZE THE TAIL AWAY FROM THE BODY – THE VEIN WILL COME WITH IT.

ASIAN VEGETABLE SALAD (0)

CORE INGREDIENT
100 gm bean sprouts

FRUIT/VEGETABLES
1 avocado, peeled and sliced
1/2 cucumber, sliced
12–16 snowpeas, halved
8–10 baby mushrooms, sliced
4–6 spring onions, sliced
1 red pepper, sliced
1 T lemon juice

FROM THE CUPBOARD
2 T olive oil
1 T soya sauce
1 T sesame seeds

HERBS AND SPICES
3 T chopped coriander
salt and pepper to taste

1 Prepare all the vegetables, and mix together in a salad bowl. (We like the snowpeas raw, but you can blanch them for about 1 minute in boiling water if you prefer)

2 Toast the sesame seeds in a small frying pan on the stove for 1–2 minutes then add to the vegetables

3 Shake the olive oil, lemon juice and soya sauce together, season to taste and pour over the salad.

This salad is delicious served with chicken burgers (page 227–8).

PREPARATION TIME: 10 mins

SALADS ARE MORE ATTRACTIVE IF THE VEGETABLES ARE CUT INTO SMALL PIECES.

AVOCADO AND PAPAYA SALAD (1)
CORE INGREDIENT
2 avocados, peeled and sliced

FRUIT/VEGETABLES
1 medium papaya, peeled, seeded and sliced
1 T lime or lemon juice
mixed green salad of rocket, watercress, baby spinach
8 cherry tomatoes, halved

FROM THE CUPBOARD
1/2 cup walnuts
2 T walnut oil
1 T red wine vinegar

HERBS AND SPICES
salt and pepper to taste

1 Toast the walnuts in the oven or in a pan then lightly chop them into small pieces
2 Arrange the mixed salad leaves on individual plates with the halved cherry tomatoes

3 Toss the avocado and papaya gently with the lemon or lime juice and place on top of the lettuce leaves
4 Whisk together the walnut oil and vinegar with salt and pepper to taste and pour over the salad
5 Sprinkle with the toasted walnuts.

PREPARATION TIME: 10 mins

VARIATIONS:
● *Use mango or rock melon instead of papaya.*
● *Serve with a few steamed, or stir-fried prawns.*

BEAN AND SPRING ONION SALAD (3)
CORE INGREDIENT
10 spring onions, chopped

FRUIT/VEGETABLES
1 red onion, chopped
120 gm olives
1 red pepper, chopped
60 gm fresh green beans, cut into 3cm pieces
2 T lemon juice

FROM THE CUPBOARD
1 cup borlotti beans
1 cup cannellini beans
1 cup red kidney beans
1 T capers
3 T olive oil
1 tsp mustard

HERBS AND SPICES
1/4 cup of fresh parsley, chopped

1 Drain and rinse the canned beans and mix them together in a serving bowl
2 Blanch the green beans, drain, cool and add to the canned beans together with the capers, olives, red peppers and spring onions
3 Whisk together the olive oil, lemon juice and mustard and pour over the beans, add the parsley and stir to mix well
4 Chill in the fridge for 30 minutes, but bring back to room temperature before serving.

PREPARATION TIME:
10 minutes

BEETROOT AND CARROT SALAD (0)
CORE INGREDIENT
1 medium raw beetroot, peeled and grated

FRUIT/VEGETABLES
4 carrots, grated
4 sticks celery, sliced
1 fennel bulb, grated

FROM THE CUPBOARD
1/4 cup olive oil
1 T red wine vinegar
1 T pine nuts

HERBS AND SPICES
salt and pepper to taste

1 Mix together the beetroot, carrot, fennel and celery
2 Toast the pine nuts for a few minutes in the oven or in a pan until they turn golden and add to the vegetables
3 Shake together the oil and vinegar, season to taste and pour over the salad.

PREPARATION TIME:
5–10 minutes

VARIATION:
● *Use red or green cabbage instead of beetroot.*

BROCCOLI AND CAULIFLOWER SALAD (0)
CORE INGREDIENT
1/2 medium-sized cauliflower, cut into florets

FRUIT/VEGETABLES
1 small head of broccoli, cut into florets

FROM THE CUPBOARD
1/4 cup olive oil
1 T red wine vinegar

HERBS AND SPICES
2 T chopped chives
2 T chopped mint
salt and pepper

1 Steam or boil the broccoli and cauliflower florets until they are just tender
2 Drain and plunge them into cold water immediately and put them into the fridge to keep crisp
3 Mix together the olive oil, vinegar and salt and pepper to taste and, just before serving, mix in the chopped herbs
4 Pour the dressing over the salad and serve.

PREPARATION TIME: 15 minutes

CARROT SALAD (1)
Contributed by Gill's dad, Peter Tidey.

CORE INGREDIENT
4 large carrots, peeled and grated (about 250 gm)

FRUIT/VEGETABLES
1/2 red onion, finely chopped
1 small orange, peeled
1 T lemon juice

FROM THE CUPBOARD
60 gm pine nuts
60 gm raisins
2 T olive oil

HERBS AND SPICES
salt and pepper to taste
2 T fresh coriander (optional)

1 Toast the pine nuts in the oven or in a frying pan on the stove until they change colour
2 Finely chop the orange and reserve any juice
3 Whisk together the olive oil, lemon juice and reserved orange juice
4 Stir the carrots, onion, orange, nuts and raisins together gently
5 Drizzle the dressing over the salad, season to taste and garnish with fresh coriander. (If the salad is too moist, drain off some of the dressing.)

PREPARATION TIME: 10 minutes

CHICKPEA WITH ROASTED VEGETABLE SALAD (3)
CORE INGREDIENT
1 can chickpeas

FRUIT/VEGETABLES
3–4 cloves garlic, minced
2 T lemon juice
2 cups roasted vegetables (page 154)
2 T lemon juice

FROM THE CUPBOARD
1/4 cup olive oil

HERBS AND SPICES
2 T chopped mint
2 T chopped parsley

1 Rinse and drain the chickpeas
2 Prepare the dressing by mixing the olive oil, garlic and lemon juice
3 Put the chickpeas in a serving bowl, stir through the roast vegetables, pour over the dressing, add plenty of mixed chopped herbs and mix carefully.

Serve by itself, or with grilled lamb chops, or chicken, or even with left-over roast lamb.

PREPARATION TIME:
5 minutes

CHICKPEA AND TOMATO SALAD (3)
CORE INGREDIENT
175 gm dried chickpeas soaked overnight or 1 can chickpeas

FRUIT/VEGETABLES
3 medium tomatoes, chopped
1 small red onion, chopped
1 green pepper, sliced
2–3 cloves garlic, crushed
1/4 cup lemon juice
1 tsp fresh minced ginger

FROM THE CUPBOARD
2 T olive oil

HERBS AND SPICES
1 T fresh chopped mint
1 red chilli, sliced

salt and pepper to taste

1 Drain dried chickpeas after soaking overnight, cover with fresh water and simmer for 2 hours, then drain and cool, or rinse canned chickpeas well, drain and pat dry with a clean cloth
2 Mix together the chickpeas, tomatoes, onion, green pepper and mint
3 Shake together the olive oil, garlic, ginger, chilli and lemon juice and season to taste
4 Pour the dressing over the salad and stir to mix thoroughly.

PREPARATION TIME:
6–8 minutes (if using canned chickpeas)

GREEN SALAD WITH COCONUT DRESSING (4)
CORE INGREDIENT
200 gm green beans

FRUIT/VEGETABLES
1/2 cucumber, sliced
1 green pepper, sliced
4–6 spring onions, chopped
1 avocado, peeled, stoned and sliced
60 gm bean sprouts
4 stalks asparagus, cut into 2 1/2 cm pieces (optional)
1 T lemon juice

FROM THE CUPBOARD
1/4 cup coconut milk
2 T olive oil

HERBS AND SPICES
2 T mint

1 Steam the beans and asparagus until they are just tender, plunge them into cold water and refrigerate to cool
2 Mix together the spring onions, green pepper, bean sprouts, chilled beans, asparagus and chopped mint
3 Peel and slice the avocado, sprinkle with lemon juice to stop it turning brown and add it to the salad
4 Shake the coconut milk and olive oil together and pour over the salad.

PREPARATION TIME: 10 mins

INDONESIAN-STYLE VEGETABLE SALAD (5)
CORE INGREDIENT
4 eggs, hard-boiled

FRUIT/VEGETABLES
1 small cauliflower
120 gm green beans
1 large carrot, julienned
2 medium potatoes
1 cucumber, julienned
150 gm bean sprouts
1 clove garlic

FROM THE CUPBOARD
150 gm peanuts
1 tsp soya sauce
1 cup coconut milk

HERBS AND SPICES
1 tsp chilli sauce

1 Peel and slice the eggs or cut them into quarters
2 Prepare all the vegetables and steam or boil them separately until they are just cooked, then plunge them into cold water and refrigerate them to keep them crisp
3 Roast the peanuts in the oven for about 5 minutes and then process with the coconut milk, garlic, soya sauce and chilli sauce to a smooth sauce
4 Arrange the vegetables in sections on a plate, add the eggs and serve with the peanut sauce.

PREPARATION TIME:
10 minutes/COOKING TIME:
15 minutes

PLUNGE HARD-BOILED
EGGS INTO COLD
WATER TO AVOID
THEM FORMING
BLACK RINGS
ROUND THE YOLKS

ITALIAN SALAD (0)
CORE INGREDIENT
5–6 vine-ripened tomatoes

FRUIT/VEGETABLES
1 small red onion, finely
  chopped
1/2 cucumber, chopped
1 stick celery, finely chopped
1 red pepper, finely chopped,
1 green pepper, finely chopped
2 cloves garlic, crushed

FROM THE CUPBOARD
1/3 cup olive oil
2 T red wine vinegar
2 thick slices stale coarse bread

HERBS AND SPICES
1/2 cup fresh basil, chopped
salt and pepper to taste

1 Remove the crusts from the
bread and tear it into pieces.
Sprinkle with cold water (do not
make it soggy)
2 Gently mix together all the
salad ingredients, bread and
basil and season to taste
3 Shake the olive oil and
vinegar together, pour over the
salad and stir to mix well
4 Allow the salad to stand for 30
minutes before serving.

PREPARATION TIME:
5–6 minutes

MARINATED MUSHROOMS (0)
CORE INGREDIENT
250 gm baby mushrooms

FRUIT/VEGETABLES
1 T lemon juice
2–3 cloves garlic, finely chopped

FROM THE CUPBOARD
1/4 cup olive oil

HERBS AND SPICES
2 T chopped parsley
salt and pepper

1 Mix all the ingredients
together thoroughly and pour
over the mushrooms
2 Stir well to ensure the
mushrooms are well coated
with the oil and leave them to
marinate overnight in the fridge.

Serve as part of an antipasto
plate with roasted vegetables
(page 154) and artichokes and
sunblush tomatoes or just add
to a green salad.

PREPARATION TIME:
5 minutes, plus overnight
marinating

MIXED GREEN SALAD (0)
CORE INGREDIENT
60 gm mixed lettuce leaves

FRUIT/VEGETABLES
60 gm rocket
60 gm baby spinach leaves
1 green pepper, sliced
1/2 cucumber, sliced
4-6 marinated artichokes
1/2 cup green grapes
1 green apple
4-6 spring onions, chopped
8-12 olives (optional)
1/2 tsp lemon juice

FROM THE CUPBOARD
3 T olive oil
1 T balsamic vinegar
1 tsp Dijon mustard

HERBS AND SPICES
1 cup mixed herbs
salt and pepper

1 Core and slice the apple and
sprinkle it with the lemon juice
2 Prepare all the salad
vegetables and fruit and mix in
a serving bowl with the apple
and chopped herbs
3 Shake together the oil, vinegar
and mustard, season to taste and
pour over the salad.

PREPARATION TIME:
5-6 minutes

PASTA SALAD (3)
CORE INGREDIENT
250 gm pasta shells

FRUIT/VEGETABLES
2 small zucchini
1 cup peas
1 red pepper, sliced
1 green pepper, sliced
60 gm rocket

FROM THE CUPBOARD
3 T olive oil
1 T red wine vinegar
1 tsp Dijon mustard

HERBS AND SPICES
1 T chopped parsley
1 T chopped basil

1 Cook the pasta in plenty of
boiling water according to the
instructions on the packet.
Drain and rinse under cold
water
2 Wash the zucchini and cut
into slices, then sauté with the
peas in one tablespoon olive oil
until they are just tender. Let
them cool before adding them to
the pasta
3 Add the peppers, rocket and
the chopped herbs to the pasta
and mix together
4 Shake together the remaining
olive oil, vinegar and mustard
and pour over the pasta and mix
gently.

PREPARATION TIME:
5-6 minutes/COOKING TIME:
10 minutes

PEAR, ARTICHOKE AND WALNUT SALAD (0)

CORE INGREDIENT
3–4 cups mixed green salad
  leaves

FRUIT/VEGETABLES
2 pears, peeled and sliced
1/2 cup green grapes
8–12 marinated artichokes,
  quartered

FROM THE CUPBOARD
100 gm fresh walnut pieces
1/4 cup walnut oil
2 T cider vinegar

HERBS AND SPICES
salt to taste
black pepper
3 T Italian parsley, chopped

1 Heat 1 tablespoon of walnut
oil and fry the walnut pieces for
2 to 3 minutes until they are
golden and crunchy, being
careful that they don't burn.
Set them aside and leave
them to cool
2 Peel and core the pears and
cut them into slices, put them
into a large bowl and grind black
pepper over them
3 Shake the remainder of the
walnut oil with the cider vinegar
and pour over the pears and
leave them to marinate for
about 30 mins

4 Prepare a mixed green salad,
add the artichokes, grapes,
walnuts, chopped parsley and
marinated pears with their
dressing, season to taste and
toss.

Serve with toasted bread
brushed with garlic and
walnut oil.

PREPARATION TIME:
5–6 minutes

*MARINATED
ARTICHOKES IN
OLIVE OIL CAN BE
FOUND IN ALL GOOD
SUPERMARKETS AND
DELICATESSENS
AND REALLY LIVEN
UP A SALAD*

PITTA BREAD SALAD (3)

Gill's friend, Diana Lampe,
introduced her to this salad,
which is absolutely delicious.

CORE INGREDIENT
1 large flat pitta bread

FRUIT/VEGETABLES
1 cucumber, chopped
3 tomatoes, chopped
6 spring onions, finely chopped
3–4 cloves garlic, crushed
3–4 T lemon juice

FROM THE CUPBOARD
1/4 cup olive oil

HERBS AND SPICES
1 cup parsley, chopped
2 T mint, chopped
3 T fresh coriander, chopped
salt and pepper

1 Put all the finely chopped
vegetables and herbs into a
serving bowl
2 Open out the pitta bread and
put it in a hot oven or under the
grill for a few minutes until it is
crisp and brown. Crumble it and
add it to the salad vegetables
and herbs
3 Shake together the olive oil
and lemon juice and pour over
the salad just before serving.

PREPARATION TIME:
6–8 minutes/COOKING TIME:
2 minutes

POTATO SALAD (3)
CORE INGREDIENT
500 gm new potatoes

FRUIT/VEGETABLES
4 spring onions, finely sliced

FROM THE CUPBOARD
1 cup plain soya 'yoghurt'
1 T olive oil

HERBS AND SPICES
salt and pepper
1 T mixed cumin, fennel and
sesame seeds

1 Boil or steam the potatoes,
then let them cool before dicing
2 Put the soya 'yoghurt' in a
bowl and lightly beat it with a
fork until it becomes 'creamy'
3 Heat the oil and lightly fry the
seeds, add them to the yoghurt,
season to taste, then gently fold
in the potatoes and the spring
onion.

PREPARATION TIME:
5–6 minutes/COOKING TIME:
15–20 minutes

VARIATION:
● *Add blanched fennel slices to*
the potatoes.

RED ONION AND TOMATO SALSA (0)
This is delicious served with roast
or barbecued leg of lamb (page
193–4) or any of the curries.

CORE INGREDIENT
3–4 medium tomatoes or 8–10
  cherry tomatoes, diced

FRUIT/VEGETABLES
1/2 large red onion, finely
  chopped
2 T lemon juice

HERBS AND SPICES
1 cup fresh coriander, chopped
1 small red chilli, chopped
1/2 tsp salt

1 Mix together the onion,
coriander, chilli and tomatoes
2 Just before serving season
with salt and pour over the
lemon juice.

PREPARATION TIME: 5 minutes

RICE AND BROCCOLI SALAD (3)
CORE INGREDIENT
2 cups cooked rice

FRUIT/VEGETABLES
250 gm broccoli florets
1 red pepper
4–6 spring onions
1 small red onion

FROM THE CUPBOARD
4 T olive oil
2 T wine vinegar
1 tsp Dijon mustard

HERBS AND SPICES
2 T chopped parsley
salt and pepper to taste

1 Steam or boil the broccoli
until it is just cooked, rinse
under cold water and refrigerate
until cool
2 Chop the red pepper, spring

onions and red onion and mix
with the rice, broccoli and
chopped parsley
3 Shake together the olive oil,
vinegar and mustard and pour
over the rice salad. Season to
taste.

PREPARATION TIME:
5–6 minutes/COOKING TIME:
15–20 minutes

RICE SALAD (3)
CORE INGREDIENT
1 cup long grain rice, washed
and drained

FRUIT/VEGETABLES
2 tomatoes, chopped
1 cucumber, cubed
5–6 spring onions, chopped
6–8 baby mushrooms, quartered
1/2 red or green pepper,
  chopped
2–3 cloves garlic, chopped
2 T lemon juice

FROM THE CUPBOARD
5 T olive oil
2 cups water

HERBS AND SPICES
1/2 tsp saffron or turmeric
2 T chopped parsley
2 T chopped mint
2 T chopped chives
salt and pepper to taste
1 red chilli, chopped (optional)

1 Heat one tablespoon of the oil, add the garlic and rice and stir-fry for 1 to 2 minutes ensuring all the rice grains are coated with oil
2 Add the water and saffron, bring to the boil, then cover and simmer for about 12 minutes until all the water has been absorbed and the rice is soft. Allow to cool
3 Add the chopped vegetables and herbs
4 Shake together the olive oil, chilli and lemon juice and pour over the salad.

PREPARATION TIME:
10 minutes

VARIATION:
● *This salad can be made with left-over steamed rice.*

ROASTED SWEET POTATO AND PUMPKIN SALAD (3)
CORE INGREDIENT
1 cup couscous

FRUIT/VEGETABLES
250 gm sweet potato
250 gm pumpkin
1 small red onion, chopped
250 gm rocket (or any mixed green salad leaves)
4 spring onions, chopped
2 T fresh lime juice

FROM THE CUPBOARD
2 T soya sauce
2 T olive oil
1 T chilli oil
2 cups vegetable stock

HERBS AND SPICES
1 red chilli, chopped
2 T mint leaves, chopped
salt
fresh parsley or coriander leaves

1 Peel the sweet potato and pumpkin and cut into cubes, place in a baking dish and drizzle with the chilli oil and a little salt. Bake in a preheated 160°C oven for about 20 minutes until the vegetables are just soft
2 Place the couscous in a bowl, pour over the boiling stock, cover and leave to stand until the stock is absorbed (about 5 minutes)
3 Add the red onion, spring onions, chilli, mint leaves and the baked pumpkin and sweet potato to the couscous and mix gently
4 Mix together the remaining oil, soya sauce and lime juice and pour over the salad
5 Garnish with parsley or coriander leaves and serve with rocket leaves.

PREPARATION TIME: 8–10 minutes/COOKING TIME: 20 minutes

SQUID SALAD (6)
CORE INGREDIENT
8 fresh baby squid, rinsed, dried and cut in half

FRUIT/VEGETABLES
120 gm mixed salad leaves
1 small cucumber, thinly sliced
1 small red onion, finely chopped
2 large field mushrooms, sliced
8–10 cherry tomatoes, halved
2 T lime or lemon juice

FROM THE CUPBOARD
4 T teriyaki marinade

HERBS AND SPICES
1 cup fresh coriander
2 tsp chilli sauce (or to taste)

1 Prepare all the salad vegetables and mix them together
2 Mix the teriyaki marinade with the chilli sauce and lime juice
3 Grill the squid in a griddle pan or under the grill or on a barbecue, for only 1 to 2 minutes each side. The tentacles may need to be cooked slightly longer. Do not be tempted to over cook them or they will be rubbery
4 Place the mixed salad on a plate, put the cooked squid on top and pour over the dressing.

PREPARATION TIME: 8–10 minutes/COOKING TIME: 4–5 minutes

THAI SALAD (0)
CORE INGREDIENT
100 gm mixed green salad leaves

FRUIT/VEGETABLES
50 gm rocket
1 red pepper, sliced
1 cup of green grapes
2 cups of beansprouts
1/2 white or orange melon, peeled and cubed
1/2 pomegranate seeds
1 T lemon juice

FROM THE CUPBOARD
2 T olive oil
1 T sesame oil
1 T soya sauce
1 T mirin

HERBS AND SPICES
2 T fresh coriander

1 Mix together all the vegetables, herbs and fruit
2 Shake together the olive and sesame oils, soya sauce, lemon juice and mirin and pour over the salad.

PREPARATION TIME:
5–10 minutes

TOMATO AND ONION SALAD (0)
CORE INGREDIENT
4 medium tomatoes, sliced

FRUIT/VEGETABLES
1 small red onion
2 spring onions, chopped

FROM THE CUPBOARD
2 T olive oil

HERBS AND SPICES
2 T fresh basil or oregano

1 Slice the tomatoes and red onion and place slices alternately on a plate
2 Sprinkle with spring onions and basil and drizzle over the olive oil.

PREPARATION TIME:
5–6 minutes

VARIATION:
● *Add black or green olives.*

WALDORF-STYLE SALAD (1)
CORE INGREDIENT
3 apples, cored and sliced

FRUIT/VEGETABLES
1 orange, peeled and chopped

6 sticks of celery, diced
4 spring onions, chopped
1 cup of mixed red and green grapes
2 T lemon juice
Cos lettuce leaves

FROM THE CUPBOARD
60 gm toasted walnuts or pine nuts
1/4 cup of raisins
1 cup of soya 'yoghurt'

HERBS AND SPICES
1 tsp black pepper

1 Toast the walnuts or pine nuts in the oven or in a frying pan on the stove and add to the bowl
2 Mix together the apple, orange, celery and spring onions in a salad bowl
3 Whisk together the yoghurt, black pepper and lemon juice and pour over the salad
4 Serve with torn lettuce leaves.

PREPARATION TIME:
10 minutes

ZUCCHINI COOKED IN RED WINE VINEGAR (3)
CORE INGREDIENT
500 gm zucchini

FRUIT/VEGETABLES
4–6 garlic cloves, minced

FROM THE CUPBOARD
1/4 cup red wine vinegar
1/4 cup lemon juice
1/2 cup olive oil

HERBS AND SPICES
salt
small bunch of mint leaves
chopped parsley

1 Wash the zucchini, cut them in half and slice thinly lengthways
2 Heat the oil and sauté the garlic for one minute, then add the zucchini, vinegar and salt and fry on a very gentle heat for about 20 to 25 minutes until the zucchini are tender but still firm
3 Put into a container, sprinkle with chopped fresh mint and parsley, cover and refrigerate overnight.

Serve at room temperature on fresh bread with hummus (page 107), or add to a salad.

PREPARATION TIME:
5 minutes/COOKING TIME:
20–25 minutes

WARM SALADS

CHICKEN AND CORIANDER SALAD (6)
CORE INGREDIENT
2 chicken breasts, sliced

FRUIT/VEGETABLES
2 vine-ripened tomatoes, sliced
2 cloves garlic, crushed
3 cups of mixed green salad leaves
4 spring onions, chopped
1 red pepper, sliced
1 cup of red and green grapes
1 T lime or lemon juice

FROM THE CUPBOARD
1 T olive oil
1 T sesame oil
3 T mirin
1 T light soya sauce
1 T sesame seeds

HERBS AND SPICES
3 T chopped fresh coriander
3 T chopped fresh mint
2 red chillies

1 Toast the sesame seeds in a dry pan for 2 to 3 minutes
2 Sprinkle the chicken with black pepper and olive oil and grill or stir-fry for 3 to 4 minutes until the chicken is cooked through
3 To make the dressing, heat the sesame oil, fry the garlic for one minute, add the soya sauce, mirin, lime or lemon juice and simmer for one minute
4 Mix together the salad leaves, tomatoes, spring onions, red pepper, grapes, coriander and mint and serve on

individual plates

5 Top with the chicken, pour over the dressing and sprinkle with toasted sesame seeds.

PREPARATION TIME:
8–10 minutes/COOKING TIME:
5–6 minutes

CHICKEN NOODLE SALAD (6)

CORE INGREDIENT
2–3 chicken breasts, sliced

FRUIT/VEGETABLES
1 T ginger, minced
4–6 spring onions chopped
1/2 cucumber, julienned
1 cup bean sprouts

FROM THE CUPBOARD
1 T olive oil
1 T sesame oil
2 T light soya sauce
330 gm fresh soba (Japanese)
  noodles

HERBS AND SPICES
2 T chopped coriander

1 Whisk together the sesame oil, ginger and soya sauce, pour over the chicken and leave to marinate for at least 30 minutes, then remove the chicken from the marinade and reserve the liquid

2 Heat the olive oil, add the

chicken and stir-fry for 3 to 4 minutes until cooked

3 Cook the noodles according to the instructions on the packet and drain

4 Add the chicken, cucumber, bean sprouts and spring onions to the noodles while they are still warm and pour over the marinade

5 Garnish with chopped coriander and serve warm or cold.

PREPARATION TIME:
5 minutes, plus marinating/
COOKING TIME: 6–8 minutes

DUCK AND ORANGE SALAD (6)

CORE INGREDIENT
2–3 duck breasts

FRUIT/VEGETABLES
500 gm baby spinach leaves
1 red pepper, sliced
1 T orange juice
1 T lemon juice
2 small mandarins

FROM THE CUPBOARD
2–3 T olive oil
1 tsp sesame oil
1 tsp soya sauce

HERBS AND SPICES
1 red chilli, chopped (optional)
black pepper

1 Slice the duck breasts and stir-fry in one to two tablespoons of olive oil for about 4 to 5 minutes
2 While the duck is cooking, stir-fry the chilli and red pepper with the remaining olive oil for 2–3 minutes in a separate frying pan
3 Add the mandarin and warm through for about 30 seconds. Add the orange juice, lemon juice, soya sauce and spinach and stir gently until the spinach begins to wilt
4 Serve on to individual plates topped with the duck and season with black pepper.

PREPARATION TIME:
5 minutes/COOKING TIME:
6–8 minutes

DUCK BREAST IN SOYA SAUCE WITH MELON SALAD (6)

CORE INGREDIENT
2–3 duck breasts, sliced

FRUIT/VEGETABLES
1 galia melon, cut into cubes
100 gm mixed green salad
50 gm watercress
1 red pepper, sliced
1–2 cloves garlic, crushed

FROM THE CUPBOARD
2 T light soya sauce
2 T olive oil

2 T dry sherry or mirin
1 T red wine vinegar
1 T sherry

HERBS AND SPICES
fresh black pepper

1 Remove the skin from the duck breasts and discard
2 Marinate the duck breasts in soya sauce for at least 2 hours
3 Heat the olive oil in a frying pan, add the duck breasts and brown each side for about 2 to 3 minutes. Lower the heat and add the remaining marinade and one tablespoon of sherry or mirin. Continue to sauté for about 4 to 5 minutes turning the duck occasionally. When cooked, place the duck breasts on a plate, pour over the juices and leave for 5 minutes
4 Mix together the green salad, watercress, red pepper and melon
5 Mix the remaining sherry, with the garlic, vinegar and olive oil and pour over the salad
6 Serve the salad on plates, add the finely sliced duck breasts and pour any remaining juices over the meat.

PREPARATION TIME:
5 minutes, plus marinating
COOKING TIME: 8–10 minutes

NICOISE SALAD WITH GRILLED CHICKEN (6)

CORE INGREDIENT
2 chicken breasts

FRUIT/VEGETABLES
2–3 cups Cos lettuce leaves
1/2 red onion, thinly sliced
100 gm green beans, cut into
2 1/2 cm pieces
1 red pepper, sliced
8–10 cherry tomatoes, halved
60 gm snowpeas, halved
12–16 baby new potatoes
2 T lemon juice
8–12 marinated artichoke
  hearts, quartered

FROM THE CUPBOARD
2 T balsamic vinegar
4 T olive oil

HERBS AND SPICES
1 tsp chilli sauce
salt and pepper to taste
2 T chopped basil or parsley

1 Cut the chicken breasts into 3 to 4 pieces and put in a bowl
2 Mix together one tablespoon of the olive oil with the balsamic vinegar and chilli sauce and pour over the chicken. Ensure the chicken pieces are well coated and leave to marinate for at least 30 minutes
3 Pour boiling water over the beans, leave them for about 5 mins, then drain, rinse under cold water and put into the fridge to cool
4 Steam or boil the potatoes until they are tender
5 Tear the lettuce leaves into pieces then add the tomatoes, artichoke hearts, chilled beans and snowpeas
6 Prepare the salad dressing by mixing together the remaining olive oil and vinegar and pour it over the salad
7 Heat the frying pan, add the chicken and the marinade and stir occasionally until the chicken is thoroughly cooked. If the marinade dries before the chicken is cooked add a little extra olive oil
8 Serve the salad in bowls with the chicken placed on top sprinkled with fresh basil or parsley.

PREPARATION TIME:
10 minutes/COOKING TIME:
6–8 minutes

VARIATION:
● *Use hard boiled eggs (5)*
instead of chicken.

POTATO AND GREEN BEAN SALAD (3)

CORE INGREDIENT
250 gm new potatoes

FRUIT/VEGETABLES
250 gm green beans
3 cloves garlic

FROM THE CUPBOARD
1/4 cup olive oil
4 T pine nuts

HERBS AND SPICES
2 cups parsley or basil
salt to taste

1 Purée the garlic, olive oil, pine nuts and basil or parsley with a pinch of salt in a food processor until it forms a coarse 'pesto'
2 Steam or boil the potatoes and green beans separately until tender
3 Drain the vegetables, mix them together and pour over the pesto while they are still hot. Serve warm.

PREPARATION TIME:
5 minutes/COOKING TIME:
15–20 minutes

VARIATION:
● *Make the pesto with coriander and walnuts.*

SPINACH AND DUCK SALAD WITH MELON (6)

CORE INGREDIENT
2–3 duck breasts

FRUIT/VEGETABLES
150 gm baby spinach leaves or mixed green salad leaves
1/4 melon, peeled and cut into slices

FROM THE CUPBOARD
2 T oyster sauce
1 T balsamic vinegar
3 T olive oil

HERBS AND SPICES
salt and pepper to taste
2 T fresh coriander, chopped

1 Make deep slashes in the duck breasts and rub in the oyster sauce. Bake on a rack in a preheated 200°C oven for 20 to 25 minutes, then slice thinly
2 Mix together the salad leaves and melon
3 Shake the oil and vinegar together, season to taste and pour over the salad. Toss and serve on individual plates
4 Top with sliced duck breasts and garnish with chopped coriander.

PREPARATION TIME:
2–3 minutes/COOKING TIME:
20–25 mins

THAI-STYLE PRAWN SALAD (6)

CORE INGREDIENT
250 gm green prawns

FRUIT/VEGETABLES
4 cloves garlic
2 cm piece (1 T) ginger
1/2 red onion, sliced
1/2 red pepper, sliced
2 T fresh lemon or lime juice
2–3 cups of mixed salad leaves
4 spring onions, chopped
8–10 cherry tomatoes
1/4 cucumber, sliced
12 fresh snowpeas

FROM THE CUPBOARD
2 T olive oil
2 T light soya sauce

HERBS AND SPICES
1 tsp chilli sauce or 1 fresh red
  chilli
1 cup fresh coriander leaves
salt and ground black pepper
  to taste

1 Prepare a salad with mixed salad leaves, red pepper, tomatoes, cucumber, snowpeas and finely chopped spring onions and arrange on individual plates
2 Put the olive oil, garlic, ginger, chilli, soya sauce, lime or lemon juice and coriander in a blender and mix to a paste
3 Heat a wok, add the paste and stir-fry for 1 to 2 minutes
4 Add the prawns and cook until they turn pink – about 2 to 3 minutes. Season to taste
5 Divide the prawns among the plates on top of the salad, pour over the dressing, and garnish with extra coriander.

PREPARATION TIME:
10 minutes/COOKING TIME:
5 minutes

VARIATION:
● *This salad can be made with squid (2) chicken (3) or left-over duck (3) or lamb (4) instead of the prawns. Steam or stir-fry the squid or chicken separately before adding to the spice mix.*

OTHER SALAD SUGGESTIONS
● Bean sprout, mushroom
and avocado (0)
● Couscous with grilled
chicken (3)
● Mandarin, cucumber
and watercress (0)
● Roast tomatoes with
asparagus and spinach (0)
● Rocket, fennel and
mushroom (0)
● Snowpea and mushroom (0)
● Spinach, tomato,
cucumber and cannellini
beans (0)

- Tomato, cucumber, red
pepper and red onion   (0)
- Lettuce, watercress,
red onion and orange   (0)
- Spinach and bean sprout   (0)
- Avocado, cucumber and
kiwifruit   (0)
- Fennel, red pepper and
olives   (0)

*EXPERIMENT WITH
HERB-INFUSED OLIVE
OILS AND SPECIALIST
VINEGARS SUCH AS
RASPBERRY VINEGAR.*

*TO ROAST TOMATOES,
CUT VINE-RIPENED
ROMA TOMATOES IN
HALF, PLACE ON A
BAKING TRAY CUT SIDE
UP, SPRINKLE WITH
OLIVE OIL, BASIL LEAVES
AND BLACK PEPPER
AND BAKE FOR ABOUT
25 MINUTES IN A
PREHEATED
180°C OVEN.*

*TO MAKE YOUR OWN
SUNBLUSH TOMATOES,
CUT VINE TOMATOES IN
HALF, SPRINKLE WITH
SALT AND MIXED HERBS
AND BAKE IN THE OVEN
ON ITS LOWEST SETTING
FOR ABOUT 4 HOURS.
PUT IN A JAR AND
COVER WITH OLIVE
OIL. THEY WILL LAST
ABOUT A WEEK IN
THE FRIDGE.*

6.3 SLICK AND FAST SNACKS AND NIBBLES

When possible make your own bread or biscuits, substituting soya 'milk' or olive oil for dairy milk or butter in available recipes. Alternatively buy Japanese rice crackers, oat cakes or crispbreads. Low-fat, lightly salted crisps made with high-quality vegetable oils are also fine for an occasional snack. Search your Chinese foodstore for interesting Asian dairy-free snacks – our local Chinese food shop now offers crispy fried seaweed, which is delicious on its own or in salads. Use freshly shelled nuts and dried fruit.

Home-made dips and spreads are a particularly good, mouth-watering alternative to cheese. Use them on bread, biscuits or as fillings on baked potatoes, or as dips for fresh vegetables such as broccoli, celery, carrot or cucumber sticks.

AUBERGINE PURÉE (3)
CORE INGREDIENT
1–2 medium to large aubergines

FRUIT/VEGETABLES
3–4 cloves garlic
2 T lemon juice

FROM THE CUPBOARD
1 T olive oil
2 T tahini paste

HERBS AND SPICES
1–2 T fresh parsley
salt and pepper
1 tsp paprika

1 Preheat the oven to 150°C and roast the whole aubergine for about 30 minutes until it has gone soft
2 Allow the aubergine to cool, remove the flesh and put it in a food processor
3 Add the garlic, olive oil, lemon juice and tahini and process to a smooth paste and season to taste (experiment and add more or less lemon juice or tahini to suit your taste)
4 Serve with chopped fresh parsley and a sprinkling of paprika.

PREPARATION TIME:
1–2 minutes/COOKING TIME:
25–30 minutes

VARIATIONS:
● Add a small roasted onion to the aubergine.
● Omit the tahini paste.

AVOCADO ON TOAST (3)

CORE INGREDIENT
1/2 ripe avocado for each slice
of bread

FRUIT/VEGETABLES
1 ripe tomato or 3–4 sundried
or sunblush tomatoes per slice
of bread
1–2 garlic cloves, peeled

FROM THE CUPBOARD
dash of balsamic vinegar
toasted organic bread

HERBS AND SPICES
salt and pepper to taste
1 tsp basil leaves, torn

1 Toast the bread and then rub
with the garlic clove
2 Peel and mash the avocado
and spread onto the toasted
bread
3 Slice the tomato, sprinkle with
a dash of balsamic vinegar and
salt and pepper to taste and put
on top of the avocado. Garnish
with torn basil leaves and serve
immediately.

PREPARATION TIME:
3–4 minutes/COOKING TIME:
2–3 mins

AVOCADO SALAD/ GUACAMOLE (0)

CORE INGREDIENT
2 avocados, roughly diced

FRUIT/VEGETABLES
1 small red onion, finely
chopped
1 large tomato, diced
1 T lime or lemon juice

FROM THE CUPBOARD
1 tsp capers (optional)

HERBS AND SPICES
1 red chilli (optional)
1 T chopped coriander
1 T chopped chives

1 Mix all the ingredients in a
bowl and serve as a salad.

PREPARATION TIME: 5–6 mins

VARIATION:
● *Leave out the capers, purée and
serve as a dip.*

BEETROOT DIP (3)

CORE INGREDIENT
500 gm beetroot

FRUIT/VEGETABLES
2 T lemon juice
3–4 cloves garlic

FROM THE CUPBOARD
2 T olive oil

HERBS AND SPICES
1/2 tsp salt
1 tsp cayenne pepper

1 Wash the beetroot and trim
the leaves (do not cut off the
tapering tail)
2 Boil in plenty of lightly salted
water for about 1 1/2 hours or
until it is tender (it can be
roasted brushed with olive oil)
3 Purée the beetroot with the
other ingredients in a food
processor until it is smooth.

PREPARATION TIME:
2–3 minutes/COOKING TIME:
1 1/2 hours

VARIATION:
● *Mix with 200 mls of soya
yoghurt.*

**CANNELLINI BEAN
DIP (3/4)**
CORE INGREDIENT
175 gm dried cannellini beans
  or 1 can

FRUIT/VEGETABLES
4–5 cloves garlic
2 T lemon juice

FROM THE CUPBOARD
2 T olive oil
2 T water

HERBS AND SPICES
2 tsp finely chopped fresh
  rosemary or mint
salt and pepper to taste

1 Soak the dried beans
overnight and drain, add to a
pan, cover them with water and
simmer in plenty of water for
about 2 hours or until they are
tender. Alternatively, rinse and
drain the canned beans
thoroughly
2 Put all the ingredients in a
food processor and blend until
smooth, add a little more water
as necessary
3 Serve drizzled with olive oil
and a sprinkle of paprika.

PREPARATION TIME:
2–3 minutes, plus overnight
soaking if using dried
beans/COOKING TIME:
2 hours if using dried beans

VARIATIONS:
● *Add one tablespoon of tomato
paste and use sage leaves instead
of the rosemary.*
● *Stir in a can of rinsed and
drained chickpeas, two
tablespoons of chopped parsley, a
little olive oil and season with lots
of black pepper.*

CARROT DIP (3)
CORE INGREDIENT
500gm carrots, scrubbed and
  coarsely chopped

FRUIT/VEGETABLES
3–4 cloves garlic
2 cm ginger

FROM THE CUPBOARD
4 T olive oil
2 T red wine vinegar

HERBS AND SPICES
1–2 tsp ground cumin
1 tsp paprika
1 tsp cayenne pepper
salt and pepper to taste
1 tsp cinnamon
2 T parsley or coriander

1 Boil or steam the carrots until
they are soft and then drain
2 Put the carrots in a food
processor with the other ingredients, except cinnamon and
parsley, and purée until smooth
3 Serve cold garnished with
sprinkled cinnamon, a drizzle of
olive oil and some chopped
fresh parsley or coriander.

PREPARATION TIME: 5 mins
COOKING TIME: 15 mins

VARIATION:
● *Use half sweet potato and half
carrot.*

CUCUMBER AND SOYA 'YOGHURT' (TZATZIKI) (1)
CORE INGREDIENT
500 gm plain soya 'yoghurt'

FRUIT/VEGETABLES
1 cucumber, peeled and
  finely chopped
1–2 cloves garlic, crushed
1 tsp lemon juice

FROM THE CUPBOARD
1 T olive oil

HERBS AND SPICES
1 tsp fine sea salt
3 T finely chopped fresh mint
black pepper

1 Put the cucumber into a
colander and sprinkle with sea
salt. Leave it to expel its water
for about 30 minutes
2 Drain the 'yoghurt' through
fine cheesecloth (optional)
3 Mix the garlic with the
'yoghurt'
4 Rinse the cucumber and dry in
kitchen paper, squeezing gently to
expel as much water as possible.
Mix gently with the 'yoghurt'
5 Add the chopped mint, a
sprinkle of black pepper and the
lemon juice and garnish with
mint sprigs.

PREPARATION TIME: 5 mins,
plus 30 mins soaking

HUMMUS (3)
CORE INGREDIENT
1 can chickpeas or 175 gm dried
  chickpeas soaked overnight
  and boiled in freshwater for
  1–2 hours

FRUIT/VEGETABLES
4 cloves garlic
3 T lemon juice

FROM THE CUPBOARD
1/3 cup tahini
1 T olive oil
1/4 – 1/2 cup of water

HERBS AND SPICES
1 tsp salt
1 tsp paprika

1 Add the chickpeas, garlic,
tahini, salt and lemon juice to a
food processor or blender and
gradually add water until the
hummus reaches a smooth
creamy consistency
2 Put in a bowl, pour a little
olive oil on the surface and
sprinkle with paprika.

PREPARATION TIME:
2 minutes/COOKING TIME: 1–2
hours if using dried chickpeas

PEPPERS WITH BALSAMIC VINEGAR (3)
CORE INGREDIENT
4 peppers (red, orange or yellow)

FROM THE CUPBOARD
2 T olive oil
1/4 cup balsamic vinegar

HERBS AND SPICES
salt and pepper to taste

1 Seed and coarsely chop the
peppers
2 Put them in a frying pan,
pour over the olive oil and
balsamic vinegar, season with
salt and pepper and cook gently
over a low heat for about 30
minutes. If they become dry add
more olive oil and balsamic
vinegar
3 Serve on toasted bread rubbed
with a garlic clove.

PREPARATION TIME:
2–3 minutes/COOKING TIME:
30 minutes

VARIATION:
● *Use onions and fry with a
teaspoon of balsamic vinegar until
they caramelise.*

SANDWICH SUGGESTIONS
● Aubergine dip with grilled
mushrooms (3)
● Roasted vegetables (3)
● Hummus with salad greens
and grilled chicken or duck (6)
● Cannellini bean dip or
hummus with grilled figs (3)
● Avocado and bacon (7)

● Cucumber and tomato (3)
● Lettuce and carrot salad (3)

SPINACH PASTIES (3)
CORE INGREDIENT
1 packet spring roll wrappers

FRUIT/VEGETABLES
500 gm spinach
1 onion, finely chopped
3–4 cloves garlic, chopped

FROM THE CUPBOARD
2 T pine nuts
2 T olive oil

HERBS AND SPICES
salt and pepper
1 tsp cayenne pepper

1 Toast the pine nuts in the oven or a small frying pan for 2 to 3 minutes, remove from the heat and leave to cool
2 Heat the oil and sauté the onion for 2 to 3 minutes then add the garlic and cayenne pepper and continue to sauté for another 1 to 2 minutes, then remove from the heat
3 Finely chop the spinach, add the pine nuts and mix with the onions and garlic
4 Make triangles as in the vegetable samosas recipe (page 109–10) and shallow fry until the pastry is golden brown.

PREPARATION TIME:
2–3 minutes, plus folding about 20 minutes/COOKING TIME:
6–8 minutes

SWEET POTATO PURÉE (3)
CORE INGREDIENT
500 gm sweet potato, cut into cubes

FRUIT/VEGETABLES
1 large onion, chopped
3–4 cloves garlic, chopped
1 T lemon juice

FROM THE CUPBOARD
3 T olive oil
2 T red wine vinegar
1/4 cup water

HERBS AND SPICES
1–2 tsp ground ginger
1 tsp paprika
1 tsp cayenne pepper
1/2 tsp turmeric
1 tsp cinnamon
salt and pepper to taste
2 T chopped parsley or coriander

1 Heat the oil and fry the onion for 2 to 3 minutes before adding the garlic, sweet potato and all the spices, except the fresh coriander or parsley, and sauté for another 1 to 2 minutes. Add the water and simmer for about 15 minutes

2 Add the lemon juice and purée to a smooth paste
3 Serve drizzled with olive oil and chopped fresh coriander.

PREPARATION TIME:
5 minutes/COOKING TIME:
20 minutes

VARIATION:
● *Serve with raisins and toasted pine nuts.*

TOMATO 'BRUSCHETTA' (3)
(per person)
CORE INGREDIENT
1 tomato

FRUIT/VEGETABLES
1 clove garlic

FROM THE CUPBOARD
1 slice toast or a muffin

HERBS AND SPICES
1 tsp olive oil
1 T chopped basil leaves

1 Toast or grill the bread
2 Peel the garlic clove and rub over the toasted bread (the toast will act as a grater)
3 Slice the tomatoes, mix with finely chopped basil leaves and toss in the olive oil
4 Serve the tomato piled on toast.

PREPARATION TIME:
2–3 minutes

VARIATIONS:
● *Replace the fresh tomatoes with sunblush tomatoes.*
● *Spread the bread with mashed avocado or hummus before putting on the tomatoes.*
● *Use black olive paste as a spread before adding the tomatoes.*

VEGETABLE SAMOSAS (3)
These are a little fiddly to make but are wonderful snacks to have with drinks. If you make a large batch you can freeze some and keep them for later. Warm them in the oven, straight from the freezer, until the pastry becomes crisp.

CORE INGREDIENT
1 packet large spring roll
  wrappers

FRUIT/VEGETABLES
1 medium onion, finely
  chopped
1 T garlic, minced
1 T ginger, minced
150 gm cauliflower, finely
  chopped
500 gm potatoes, diced
1 cup frozen peas
1 cup frozen corn
1T lemon juice

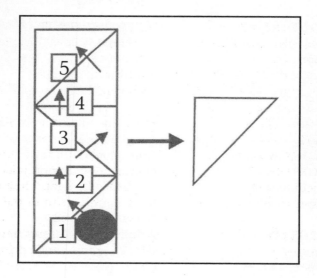

FROM THE CUPBOARD
2 T peanut or sunflower oil
1/2 cup water

HERBS AND SPICES
1 red chilli or 1 tsp cayenne
   pepper
1 tsp turmeric
2 tsp cumin
1 tsp salt
3 T fresh coriander and
   mint, chopped

1 Heat the oil, fry the onion for
2 to 3 minutes then add the
garlic, ginger and spices and
stir-fry for another 1 to 2
minutes
2 Add the potatoes and water
and simmer for about 10
minutes until the potatoes are
just tender
3 Turn off the heat and add the
cauliflower, peas, corn,
coriander and mint, mix
thoroughly and leave to cool
4 Thaw the pastry and cut the
squares into three slices
vertically *(see diagram above)*
5 Peel off a single piece of
pastry, add a heaped
teaspoonful of the vegetable
mixture into the bottom right-
hand corner of the pastry and
keep folding the pastry until it
forms a triangle
6 Shallow fry the samosas in
sunflower oil and turn until
both sides are golden brown.

Serve with chilli dipping sauce
or soya sauce or coriander pesto.

PREPARATION TIME:
10 minutes, plus cooling and
folding approximately 20
minutes/COOKING TIME:
15 minutes, plus 2–3 minutes
frying

VIETNAMESE VEGETABLE AND PRAWN ROLLS (6)
CORE INGREDIENT
500 gm medium prawns
1 packet spring roll wrappers

FRUIT/VEGETABLES
1 medium carrot
1 red pepper
2 cm fresh ginger, slivered
60 gm bean sprouts
4 spring onions
1T lemon juice
1T ginger, minced

FROM THE CUPBOARD
1 T olive oil for marinade
olive or sunflower oil for
   shallow frying rolls

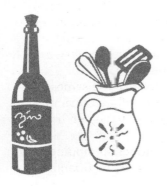

HERBS AND SPICES
2 long red chillies (or to taste)
coriander sprigs
mint leaves, chopped
60 gm chives, halved

1 Marinate the prawns for at
least 2 to 3 hours with one
tablespoon of olive oil, one
tablespoon of lemon juice and
the minced ginger. Then stir-fry
for 3–4 minutes until the
prawns turn pink
2 Julienne the carrot, red
pepper, chillies and spring
onions and mix with the bean
sprouts, coriander leaves, mint
and chives
3 On a spring roll wrapper,
across a diagonal corner, put a
handful of the vegetable mix
and 2 to 3 prawns. Roll wrapper
halfway, fold in the corners
and continue to roll up.
Shallow fry in hot olive or
sunflower oil for 2 to 3 minutes
until the wrappers are golden
brown
4 Serve with chilli or soya
sauce or Thai chilli dipping
sauce.

PREPARATION TIME: 15–20
mins, plus 2 hours marinating
COOKING TIME: 3–4 minutes
SHORT CUT: Cooking prawns
takes only a few minutes and
they taste so much better than

pre-cooked ones. If you use pre-cooked prawns omit stage 1 and add slivers of ginger to the vegetable mix.

VARIATIONS:
● *If you don't like prawns, substitute fresh crab or any other seafood or have the vegetables on their own*
● *Use rice paper wrappers, moisten in water, pat dry and roll around the vegetables*
● *Omit the wrappers and eat as a salad with your favourite dressing.*

WALNUT DIP (1)
CORE INGREDIENT
100 gm walnut pieces

FRUIT/VEGETABLES
1 T lemon juice
3–4 garlic cloves

FROM THE CUPBOARD
1/3 cup olive oil
1 T walnut oil

HERBS AND SPICES
1 tsp cayenne pepper
1 tsp ground cumin
salt to taste
1 tsp black pepper

1 Put all the ingredients in a food processor and blend until smooth.

PREPARATION TIME:
2–3 minutes

VARIATION:
● *Add 2 tablespoons of tahini to the walnut paste to make the dip 'creamier'.*

ZUCCHINI DIP (3)
CORE INGREDIENT
3 medium zucchini, sliced

FRUIT/VEGETABLES
3–4 cloves garlic, chopped
2 T lemon juice

FROM THE CUPBOARD
3 T olive oil

HERBS AND SPICES
1/2 tsp ground cumin
1/4 tsp cayenne pepper
salt to taste

1 Heat the olive oil and gently fry the garlic and zucchini until soft
2 Put the zucchini in a food processor with a little of the oil in which it was cooked
3 Add the lemon juice, cumin, salt and chilli powder and process until it becomes smooth.

PREPARATION TIME:
2–3 minutes/COOKING TIME:
15 minutes

7 Meals to live for

HEALTHY, TEMPTING AND DELICIOUS MAIN COURSES, DESSERTS AND MEALS FOR SPECIAL OCCASIONS

- *Less than 25% of the entire meal should comprise animal protein*
- *Lightly cooked vegetables*
- *Thoroughly cooked meat and fish*
- *Mostly fruit for dessert*

Many of your favourite recipes such as roasts, grills or casseroles can be made healthier just by substituting olive oil or pure soya spread for butter or other animal fats such as lard. Use onions, lemons or peeled chestnuts to stuff poultry. Make your gravy with an organic stock cube and the water the vegetables have been cooked in. If you like cauliflower cheese, or butter on your vegetables, replace with a dollop of hummus or some other dip.

Choose salads, soups or even egg dishes from the other sections to complement these meals and turn them into a full or light dinner.

Many of the recipes in this section can be modified by leaving out animal products and substituting bean curd (tofu). To ensure adequate protein, serve with additional pulses and cereals.

SOYA CAN REPLACE MANY OF THE CORE INGREDIENTS IN THESE RECIPES. TO MAKE SURE THAT IT IS TASTY, MARINATE IT IN THE SAUCE INGREDIENTS FOR AT LEAST TWO HOURS BEFORE COOKING.

● *PEEL A WHOLE GARLIC BULB AND KEEP*
THE CLOVES IN THE FRIDGE UNTIL NEEDED –
THEY WILL LAST ABOUT A WEEK
● *TWIST GARLIC CLOVES TO PEEL OFF THEIR SKIN*
● *FREEZE CHOPPED GINGER*
● *DON'T COOK SOYA SAUCE FOR TOO LONG.*
ADD TO A DISH JUST BEFORE SERVING
● *RUBBING A PEELED GARLIC CLOVE OVER TOAST*
GIVES LOTS OF FLAVOUR BECAUSE THE TOAST
ACTS AS A GRATER
● *ALWAYS FRY ONION BEFORE ADDING GARLIC OR THE*
GARLIC WILL BURN BEFORE THE ONION IS COOKED
● *FREEZE WHOLE CHILLIES AND CHOP BEFORE*
THEY ARE COMPLETELY THAWED
● *FREEZE HERBS SUCH AS FRESH BAY LEAVES,*
LIME LEAVES AND LEMON GRASS
● *KEEP CORIANDER IN A JUG OF WATER IN*
THE FRIDGE TO MAKE IT LAST LONGER.

Always assemble all the ingredients before you start cooking,
because the cooking time for most of the meals is very short.

7.1 GREAT GRAINS (PASTA, NOODLES, RICE, AND OTHER GRAINS)

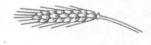

Pasta, rice, noodles and grains can be used as a basis for meals that
are inexpensive, quick, simple, tasty and healthy. Together with nuts
they are the most important source of protein in vegan diets and are
key foods for those with active cancer.

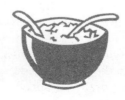

LINGUINE WITH STIR-FRIED VEGETABLES AND PRAWNS (6)

CORE INGREDIENT
200 gm fresh linguini
12–16 king prawns

FRUIT/VEGETABLES
1 onion, sliced
1 T ginger, minced
2–3 cloves garlic, minced
1 red onion, chopped
60 gm green beans
1 red pepper, chopped
60 gm fresh baby corn, halved
2 cups fresh spinach
12 chestnut mushrooms
4–5 spring onions, chopped
1 T lemon or lime juice

FROM THE CUPBOARD
2 T olive oil
1 T fish sauce
1 T soya sauce
2 T oyster sauce
1/4 cup of water

HERBS AND SPICES
1 small green Thai chilli, chopped
1 stalk lemon grass, chopped
1 tsp black pepper
2 T chopped coriander

1 Peel and de-vein the prawns leaving on the tail
2 Cook the pasta in plenty of boiling water according to the instructions on the packet, drain and set to one side
3 Stir-fry the onion in the oil for 2 to 3 mins, then add the ginger, chilli, lemon grass, corn, red pepper, beans and stir-fry for another minute
4 Add the water, cover and simmer briskly for 2 to 3 minutes
5 Add the prawns and mushrooms, cover and continue to cook for 2 to 3 minutes until the prawns turn pink
6 Add the noodles, fish sauce, soya sauce, oyster sauce and spring onions, stir through and continue to cook for another minute
7 Add the coriander and lime juice, stir through, season to taste and serve.

PREPARATION TIME:
7–8 minutes/COOKING TIME:
10 minutes

PASTA WITH ANCHOVY AND CAPER SAUCE (6)

CORE INGREDIENT
200 gm dried spaghetti
8–12 pickled anchovies from
  your local delicatessen

FRUIT/VEGETABLES
3–4 cloves garlic, chopped
4–6 spring onions, chopped
8–12 sundried/blushed tomatoes
4 medium zucchini, thickly
  sliced

FROM THE CUPBOARD
2 T small capers
4 T olive oil

HERBS AND SPICES
4 T chopped mint and
  wide-leafed parsley

1 Boil the spaghetti according to
the instructions on the packet
2 Heat 3 tablespoons of oil and
stir-fry the garlic for 1 minute
3 Add the zucchini and sauté for
about 5 to 7 minutes while the
pasta finishes cooking
4 Process or finely chop the
anchovies and capers with a
little olive oil
5 Add the anchovy and caper
mix to the zucchini, then the
spring onions, tomatoes, mint
and parsley and sauté for 1 to 2
minutes
6 Drain the pasta, add the sauce
and serve.

PREPARATION TIME:
3–4 minutes/COOKING TIME:
10 minutes

VARIATION:
● *For a spicier flavour add one or
two red chillies.*

PASTA WITH SPINACH, TOMATO AND PEAS (3)

CORE INGREDIENT
500 gm pasta such as spaghetti
or linguine

FRUIT/VEGETABLES
3–4 cloves garlic, chopped
10–12 cherry tomatoes, halved
100 gm shelled peas or one cup
  of frozen peas
1/2 medium red onion, chopped
1/2 red pepper, chopped
3 cups of spinach
6–8 marinated artichoke hearts

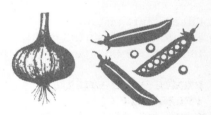

FROM THE CUPBOARD
2 T olive oil
1/4 of cup water

HERBS AND SPICES
2 T basil, finely chopped
1 tsp fresh rosemary, finely
  chopped
6–8 fresh sage leaves, finely
  chopped
salt and pepper to taste

1 Bring a large pan of water to
the boil, add the pasta and cook
according to the instructions

2 Heat the oil in a wok, and stir-fry the onion for 2 to 3 minutes
3 Add the garlic, red pepper and peas (if fresh) and stir-fry for another 1 to 2 minutes, then add the cherry tomatoes and the water and continue to cook for a further 1 to 2 minutes
4 Add the spinach, artichokes and peas (if frozen). Cook until the spinach has just wilted
5 Drain the pasta, pour over the sauce and garnish with the herbs.

PREPARATION TIME:
5 minutes/COOKING TIME:
10 minutes

PENNE WITH GREEN VEGETABLES (3)
CORE INGREDIENT
500 gm dried penne

FRUIT/VEGETABLES
4 garlic cloves, minced
350 gm broccoli, chopped
1 green pepper, chopped
60 gm snowpeas

FROM THE CUPBOARD
2 T olive oil
1/2 cup water
3-4 T pesto
8-12 kalamata olives, chopped

HERBS AND SPICES
salt and freshly ground black pepper to taste

1 Boil about 1 1/2 litres of water, add salt to taste and, when boiling strongly, add the pasta
2 At the same time heat the olive oil in a sauté pan with a lid and stir-fry the garlic for about 1 minute
3 Add the broccoli and green pepper and stir-fry for another 2 to 3 minutes. Add the water, cover and simmer for about 5 minutes
4 Turn off the heat, add the snowpeas and the olives and replace the lid. Just before serving add the pesto and stir
5 When the pasta is done (usually between 10 to 15 minutes) drain and serve in individual bowls
6 Serve the vegetables on top of the pasta and garnish with 2 to 3 sunblush or sundried tomatoes.

PREPARATION TIME:
5 minutes/COOKING TIME:
10-15 minutes

VARIATIONS:
● *Replace the pepper with asparagus, but add it 3 minutes after adding the broccoli.*
● *Add some green prawns when you add the water.*

**TO MAKE PESTO BLEND
¹/₄ – ¹/₂ CUP OF OLIVE OIL
WITH ¹/₂ CUP PINE NUTS,
2–3 GARLIC CLOVES AND
2 CUPS BASIL LEAVES, OR
PARSLEY IN A FOOD
PROCESSOR UNTIL
IT FORMS A SMOOTH
PASTE.**

PENNE WITH ZUCCHINI, CARROTS AND BASIL (3)
CORE INGREDIENT
500 gm penne

FRUIT/VEGETABLES
500 gm zucchini, sliced
4 medium carrots, sliced
1 small onion, chopped
3–4 cloves garlic, chopped

FROM THE CUPBOARD
3 T olive oil

HERBS AND SPICES
1 red chilli, sliced
1 T chopped chives
1 T chopped basil
salt and pepper to taste

1 Boil the water, add the penne and boil until it is cooked according to the packet instructions – usually around 15 minutes
2 Heat the oil in a saucepan, add the onion and sauté for about 3 to 4 minutes until it

begins to turn brown. Add the garlic and chilli and continue stirring for another 1 to 2 minutes
3 Add the carrots and continue sautéing for another 5 to 6 minutes, stirring occasionally
4 Add the zucchini and continue to sauté turning the vegetables occasionally until the zucchini are soft
5 Add the chives and basil, season to taste and mix well
6 Drain the pasta, pour over the vegetables with any olive oil remaining and serve. If necessary add another tablespoon of olive oil to ensure all the pasta is coated.

PREPARATION TIME:
7–8 minutes/COOKING TIME:
15 minutes

SPAGHETTI WITH CHERRY TOMATOES AND SNOWPEAS (3)
CORE INGREDIENT
240 gm spaghetti or linguini

FRUIT/VEGETABLES
4 cloves garlic, chopped
8–12 cherry tomatoes, halved
100 gm snowpeas, halved

FROM THE CUPBOARD
4 T olive oil

HERBS AND SPICES
20 gm fresh basil or any mixture
of fresh herbs

1 Boil the spaghetti in plenty of
boiling salted water according to
the instructions on the packet
2 About five minutes before the
spaghetti is due to be cooked,
heat 2 tablespoons of the olive
oil in a frying pan and sauté the
garlic for about 1 minute
3 Add the tomatoes and sauté
for another minute, then add
the snowpeas and continue
sautéing for another minute,
and stir in the finely chopped
basil
4 Drain the spaghetti, stir in the
pasta sauce and serve.

PREPARATION TIME:
5 minutes/COOKING TIME:
5–10 minutes

**SPAGHETTI WITH HOME-
MADE TOMATO SAUCE (3)**
CORE INGREDIENT
450 gm vine-ripened tomatoes,
finely chopped (about 6–8
medium tomatoes)
450 gm dried pasta

FRUIT/VEGETABLES
1 red onion, finely chopped
2–3 cloves garlic, minced

FROM THE CUPBOARD
2 T olive oil
1 cup red wine
1 T tomato paste

HERBS AND SPICES
salt and pepper to taste
1 red chilli (optional)
2 T chopped chives
2 T chopped parsley or basil
or oregano or a mixture

1 Cook the pasta in plenty of
boiling water according to the
instructions on the packet
2 Heat the olive oil in a large
sauté pan, add the onion and
sauté for 2 to 3 minutes then
add the garlic and chilli and
stir-fry for about 1 minute
3 Add the tomatoes, tomato
paste, wine, herbs, salt and
pepper and simmer gently for
about 30 minutes, stirring
occasionally and mashing the
tomato to a pulp using the back
of the spoon
4 Season to taste and stir in
chopped chives and parsley,
basil or oregano.

PREPARATION TIME:
7–8 minutes/COOKING TIME:
30 minutes
This sauce will keep in the
freezer for 2 to 3 months.

VARIATIONS:
● *Add one tablespoon of drained capers and 12 chopped black olives.*
● *Add 1 cup of peas and half a chopped green or red pepper.*
● *Add chopped aubergine and red peppers.*

PASTA SUGGESTIONS
● Fresh pasta with tomato, red onion and rocket
● Pasta with roast vegetables
● Linguine with onion, fennel and olives
● Spaghetti with spinach and pine nuts
● Tagliatelle with seared tuna and spicy tomato sauce.

RICE NOODLES WITH SESAME PRAWNS (6)
CORE INGREDIENTS
250 gm medium green prawns, shelled but with tail on
250 gm vermicelli rice noodles

FRUIT/VEGETABLES
2 cloves garlic, finely chopped
2 cups rocket

FROM THE CUPBOARD
1 T olive oil
1/3 cup pickled ginger, finely chopped
2 T soya sauce
1 T sesame oil
2 T sesame seeds

HERBS AND SPICES
2 T chopped coriander
1 tsp chilli sauce (optional)

1 Pour boiling water over the noodles and leave them to stand for 2 to 3 minutes until cooked, then drain and put in a serving bowl
2 Briefly toast the sesame seeds in a dry pan and add them to the noodles
3 Heat the olive oil and stir-fry the garlic, chilli and prawns for 2 to 3 minutes until the prawns turn pink
4 Add the rocket and finely chopped pickled ginger to the noodles. Mix together the sesame oil and soya sauce, pour over the noodles and mix it all together well
5 Serve with the prawns and garnish with chopped coriander.

PREPARATION TIME:
2–3 minutes/COOKING TIME:
7–8 minutes

RICE NOODLES WITH STIR-FRIED VEGETABLES (3)
CORE INGREDIENT
250 gm dried rice noodles

FRUIT/VEGETABLES
1 red onion, coarsely chopped
1 T ginger, minced

2–3 cloves garlic, minced
1 red pepper, chopped
60 gm fresh baby corn, halved
1 cup of frozen peas
2 cups of fresh spinach
8 large fresh shitake
  mushrooms, sliced
4–5 spring onions, sliced
1 T lime juice

FROM THE CUPBOARD
2 T olive oil
1 T fish sauce
1 T soya sauce
1 T oyster sauce
1/4 cup of water

HERBS AND SPICES
1 small red chilli, sliced
1 stalk lemon grass, sliced
3–4 lime leaves
black pepper to taste
2 T fresh coriander, chopped

1 Pour boiling water over the rice noodles, leave for about 3 to 4 minutes then drain and set aside
2 Heat the oil and stir-fry the onion for 2 to 3 minutes
3 Add the ginger, garlic, chilli, lemon grass, lime leaves, red pepper, mushrooms, peas and corn and stir-fry for 1 to 2 minutes
4 Add the spinach, soya sauce, oyster sauce and water, cover and simmer for 1 to 2 minutes

5 Add the noodles, spring onions and fish sauce and continue to cook for another minute
6 Stir in the lime juice and coriander and serve with freshly ground pepper to taste.

PREPARATION TIME:
7–8 minutes/COOKING TIME:
5–6 minutes

RICE VERMICELLI WITH STIR-FRIED CHICKEN (6)
CORE INGREDIENT
2–3 chicken breasts, sliced

FRUIT/VEGETABLES
4–6 cloves garlic, minced
1 T ginger, minced
12–16 asparagus spears, cut into
  5 cm lengths
6–8 oyster mushrooms, halved
6 spring onions, chopped

FROM THE CUPBOARD
500 gm rice vermicelli
2 tsp sesame oil
2 T olive oil
1 T light soya sauce
1/3 cup of water

HERBS AND SPICES
1 cup fresh coriander, chopped
1 tsp chilli sauce or to taste

1 Boil a kettle of water
2 Heat the olive oil in a wok

and sauté the garlic, ginger, chilli sauce and sliced chicken pieces for 2 to 3 minutes until the chicken pieces have changed colour

3 Add the asparagus and mushrooms, stir-fry for another minute and then add 1/3 cup of water. Cover the pan and cook slowly for another 3 to 4 minutes until the chicken pieces are cooked through

4 At this stage pour the boiling water over the rice vermicelli and leave it to soak for 2 to 3 minutes until it is soft

5 Add the sesame oil and soya sauce to the wok and stir and cook for about another minute

6 Drain the vermicelli, serve into bowls and add the chicken and vegetables. Garnish with fresh coriander and chopped spring onions, and serve with chilli sauce in separate bowls.

PREPARATION TIME:
8–10 minutes/COOKING TIME:
10–12 minutes

VARIATION:

● *Use prawns instead of chicken, but add them with the asparagus and mushrooms*

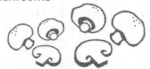

JAPANESE NOODLE SALAD (6)

CORE INGREDIENT
2–3 chicken breasts

FRUIT/VEGETABLES
2 cm ginger
3–4 garlic cloves
6 spring onions, chopped
1/2 cucumber, julienned
150 gm bean sprouts

FROM THE CUPBOARD
1 T tsp sesame oil
1 T light soya sauce
1 T mirin
330 gm fresh soba (Japanese) noodles

HERBS AND SPICES
2 T chopped coriander

1 Cook the noodles according to the instructions on the packet

2 Steam, poach or stir-fry the chicken or use left-over roast chicken

3 Process together the garlic, ginger, sesame oil, mirin and soya sauce

4 Drain the noodles, add the cucumber, bean sprouts and spring onions. Pour over the dressing, toss, and allow to cool

5 Serve with the chicken and chopped coriander.

PREPARATION TIME:
5–6 minutes/COOKING TIME:
5 minutes (15 minutes if the
chicken is uncooked)

THAI NOODLES (6)

CORE INGREDIENT
12 medium green prawns,
  shelled but with tail on
100 gm tofu, cubed
1 chicken breast, cubed

FRUIT/VEGETABLES
100 gm bean sprouts
2 shallots, chopped
4 spring onions, chopped
2 T lime or lemon juice
3–4 cloves garlic, minced
1 T ginger, minced
60 gm snowpeas, halved

FROM THE CUPBOARD
1 T fish sauce
3 T soya sauce
350 gm rice noodles
2 T olive oil
1/2 cup of roasted sesame seeds

HERBS AND SPICES
2 fresh red chillies, chopped
1 cup fresh Thai basil and mint,
  chopped
black pepper

1 Heat a pan, add the sesame
seeds and toast for 1 to 2
minutes tossing the seeds to
stop them burning. They will
continue to cook after you turn
off the heat, so turn it off in
good time
2 Break the uncooked noodles
into finger-length pieces, pour
boiling water over them, and
leave them until they become
soft, drain, and keep them warm
3 Heat the oil and add the
garlic, ginger and chillies and
stir-fry for 1 to 2 minutes
4 Add the chicken and cook for
about 3 minutes until the
chicken is cooked through
5 Add the soya sauce, fish sauce
and prawns and cook for
another 3 to 4 minutes, until the
prawns turn pink
6 Finally add the tofu, bean
sprouts, spring onions,
snowpeas and lime juice, and
continue to cook for 1–2
minutes
7 Stir through the noodles, fresh
basil and mint leaves
8 Serve with chilli and soya
sauce on the side and lemon or
lime wedges.

PREPARATION TIME:
6–8 minutes/COOKING TIME:
10 minutes

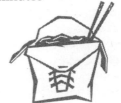

VEGETABLE NOODLES (3)

CORE INGREDIENT
400 gm fresh egg noodles
  or pasta

FRUIT/VEGETABLES
3–4 cloves garlic, chopped
1 cup of cauliflower, cut into
  small florets
1/2 cup of broccoli, cut into
  small florets
1 carrot, sliced
1 cup of Chinese or Savoy
  cabbage, chopped
1 cup of bean sprouts
1 cup of button mushrooms

FROM THE CUPBOARD
2 T olive oil
2 cups of vegetable stock
2 T soya sauce
1 T oyster sauce
1 T mirin

HERBS AND SPICES
1 red chilli (optional)

1 Cook the noodles according to
the instructions on the packet,
drain and set aside
2 Heat the oil in a wok and stir-
fry the garlic and chilli for one
minute; add the stock, oyster
sauce, soya sauce, mirin,
cauliflower, broccoli, carrot and
cabbage, cover and cook for 3 to
4 minutes
3 Add the noodles and

mushrooms, stir through and
continue to cook for 2 to 3
minutes
4 Add the bean sprouts and
continue to cook for another
minute.

PREPARATION TIME:
10 minutes/COOKING TIME:
10 minutes

COOKING BASMATI RICE

● *1 CUP OF RICE, ADD
2 CUPS OF WATER, OR*
● *2 CUPS OF RICE, ADD
3 CUPS OF WATER, OR*
● *3 CUPS OF RICE, ADD
4 CUPS OF WATER
RINSE THE RICE WELL.
ADD RICE, WATER AND A
PINCH OF SALT TO A
SAUCEPAN, BRING TO THE
BOIL, COVER AND
SIMMER FOR ABOUT 12
MINUTES – UNTIL ALL
THE WATER IS ABSORBED
AND THE RICE COOKED.*

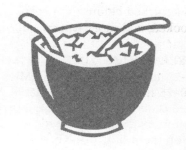

COCONUT RICE (4)

CORE INGREDIENT
2 cups basmati rice

FRUIT/VEGETABLES
1 onion, sliced
1 T ginger, minced

FROM THE CUPBOARD
2 T olive oil
3 cups coconut milk
1/2 –1 cup water

HERBS AND SPICES
1/4 tsp salt

1 Wash the rice thoroughly and drain
2 Heat the oil in a saucepan, add the onion and stir-fry for 2 to 3 minutes until the onion becomes soft
3 Add the rice, coconut milk, water and salt
4 Bring to the boil then turn down the heat as low as possible and cook covered until the liquid has been absorbed and the rice is cooked (if the liquid is absorbed before the rice is cooked, add more water).

PREPARATION TIME:
1–2 minutes/COOKING TIME:
20–25 mins

FRIED RICE (6)

Anything goes in fried rice – it is a very good dish to use up left-over rice and vegetables.

CORE INGREDIENT
60 gm small prawns/shrimps
2 chicken thighs
1–2 eggs (optional)

FRUIT/VEGETABLES
2–3 spring onions, finely sliced
1 cup of peas
1 cup of bean sprouts
1/2 cup of bamboo shoots
3–4 cloves garlic, chopped
1 small onion, chopped

FROM THE CUPBOARD
2 cups of cooked basmati rice
2 T olive or peanut oil
1 tsp sesame oil
1 T light soya sauce
1/2 cup of peanuts

HERBS AND SPICES
salt and pepper
1 red and 1 green chilli,
  chopped (optional)
2 T chopped coriander

1 If using uncooked rice, cook according to the instructions on page 124
2 Steam or stir-fry the chicken thighs or dice any left-over cooked chicken
3 Heat 1/2 tablespoon of the oil

in a frying pan, lightly beat the eggs and add to the pan. Cook as an omelette until the underside is done, turn and continue cooking until it is just set, then remove from the pan and set aside. When it is cool cut it into small strips

4 Fry or steam the prawns for a few minutes until they turn pink and put to one side – do not overcook or they will be tough and tasteless

5 In a wok, heat the remainder of the olive oil, and stir-fry the onion for 2 to 3 minutes. Add the garlic, chilli, bamboo shoots and peas, and stir-fry for 1 to 2 minutes

6 Add the cooked rice, chicken and sesame oil and all the other ingredients except the coriander and soya sauce and stir-fry until it is warmed through

7 Add the prawns, bean sprouts and soya sauce and stir through and continue to cook for 1 to 2 minutes

8 Serve garnished with plenty of coriander and extra soya and chilli sauce.

PREPARATION TIME:
5–6 minutes/COOKING TIME:
15 minutes

VEGETABLE SUSHI (3)

This is a traditional Japanese dish that often contains raw tuna, but this version uses only vegetables.

CORE INGREDIENT
2 1/2 cups sushi rice or short grain rice

FRUIT/VEGETABLES
1 cucumber
2 carrots
1 avocado

FROM THE CUPBOARD
2 1/2 cups cold water
4 T rice vinegar
3 T sugar
2 T mirin
2 T pickled red ginger
2 tsp wasabi paste
1 packet nori (Japanese seaweed, pressed into sheets)

HERBS AND SPICES
2 tsp salt

1 Wash the rice several times in cold water and leave it to drain until it is quite dry

2 Put the rice in a saucepan with the water, and bring it to the boil quickly; cover and simmer on a low heat for 15 minutes. Remove from the heat with the lid on and leave it to stand for another 10 minutes

3 Mix together the vinegar, sugar, mirin and salt, ensuring the sugar is dissolved

4 Pour the mixture over the rice, mix thoroughly and put it into the fridge to chill quickly. Stir occasionally to release heat (alternatively, you could fan it, Japanese style)

5 Cut the cucumber and carrot into long thin strips, cut the pickled ginger into strips, and peel, stone and cut the avocado into thin long strips

6 Holding a sheet of nori with a pair of tongs, wave it very briefly over a flame until it turns colour

7 Place the nori on a Japanese bamboo mat, add about half a cup of the rice and spread it over about 2/3 of the nori closest to you pressing it down firmly with your hands

8 Make a groove crossways through the middle of the rice and lay out the vegetables, the pickled ginger and a thin strip of wasabi paste in the groove

9 Push the mat over the vegetables to form a rice roll and press firmly to seal the two edges

10 Cut into pieces with a sharp moistened knife.

PREPARATION TIME: 30 minutes/COOKING TIME: 25 minutes

TOMATO RICE (3)
CORE INGREDIENT
2 cups Basmati rice

FRUIT/VEGETABLES
1 onion, sliced
3½ cups of tomato juice
2 cm ginger, minced
2–3 garlic cloves, chopped

FROM THE CUPBOARD
4 T olive oil
2 T sultanas
2 T cashew nuts

HERBS AND SPICES
½ tsp salt
4 cloves
6 whole black peppercorns
2 bay leaf

1 Wash the rice thoroughly and drain

2 Heat the oil in a wok or frying pan; fry the onions, cloves, bay leaves and peppercorns for 3 minutes then add the ginger and garlic and continue frying for 1 to 2 minutes

3 Add the rice and fry for 3 to 4 minutes

4 Add the tomato juice and salt; bring to the boil, cover the pan, turn down the heat and simmer

gently, until the rice is cooked
5 Just before serving, lightly fry
the sultanas and cashew nuts in
a little olive oil and sprinkle
over the rice.

PREPARATION TIME:
2–3 minutes/COOKING TIME:
30 minutes

PAELLA (6)
CORE INGREDIENT
2 chicken breasts
8 large tiger prawns
350 gm mussels or mixed
  seafood

FRUIT/VEGETABLES
1 small onion, chopped
4–6 cloves garlic, chopped
1/2 red pepper, seeded and
  chopped
1/2 green pepper, seeded and
  chopped
8 artichoke hearts, halved
1 cup frozen peas
1 cup frozen corn
8–10 cherry tomatoes
12 snowpeas
1 lemon, cut into wedges

FROM THE CUPBOARD
1 cup arborio rice
2 cups chicken stock
3 T olive oil

HERBS AND SPICES
1 red chilli, chopped (or to taste)

1 tsp turmeric
2 tsp paprika
2 T chopped
coriander or parsley
salt and pepper to taste

1 Heat the oil, add the chicken
breasts and sauté over a
medium heat until the chicken
is browned, remove from the
pan and cut into bite-size pieces
2 Add the onion to the same
pan and fry for 3 to 4 minutes,
then add the garlic and chilli
and continue frying for another
minute
3 Add the rice, turmeric and
peppers, stir to ensure that the
ingredients are coated with the
oil and fry for about another
minute, then add the stock.
Cover and simmer for about 8
to 9 minutes
4 Add the chicken, peas, corn,
tomatoes, prawns and mussels;
cover and continue cooking for
another 3 to 4 minutes; then add
the snowpeas and paprika, mix
together and continue to cook
for another 1 to 2 minutes. The
rice should be soft but still moist
5 Season to taste and serve with
lemon wedges and chopped
coriander or parsley.

PREPARATION TIME:
10 minutes/COOKING TIME:
30 minutes

MUSHROOM RISOTTO (3)

Marcella Hazan advises that stock is the best liquid in which to cook all risotto, except a seafood risotto, where it is best made with plain water. She also says that the best type of risotto rice to use is Carnaroli.

CORE INGREDIENT
4 Portobello mushrooms

FRUIT/VEGETABLES
8–12 dried shitake mushrooms
1 onion, chopped
2–3 cloves garlic, chopped
2 T lemon juice

FROM THE CUPBOARD
2 T olive oil
2 cups vegetable or chicken
  stock
1 cup of white wine (or extra
  stock)
1½ cups arborio rice

HERBS AND SPICES
Basil or parsley pesto
  (see page 118)

1 Soak the shitake mushrooms in 1 cup of boiling water and set aside for about 30 minutes; drain and reserve the liquid; cut the mushrooms in half or quarters
2 Sauté the olive oil and the onion for 2 to 3 minutes in a heavy-bottomed pan; then add the garlic, shitake mushrooms and rice and continue to sauté for 1 to 2 minutes stirring to ensure the rice is coated with the oil
3 Gradually add the stock, the water from the mushrooms and the wine to the rice, stirring frequently to stop the rice burning, and cook on a low heat until the rice is soft (about 20 minutes)
4 When it is cooked stir in an extra tablespoon of olive oil and the lemon juice to give it a 'creamy' texture
5 While the rice is cooking, brush the Portobello mushrooms with the pesto, grill until soft and serve on top of the risotto with extra basil or parsley.

PREPARATION TIME:
2–3 minutes, plus 30 minutes soaking/COOKING TIME:
25 minutes

VARIATION:
● *Add 2 T tomato paste and sauté with the garlic; also use red rather than white wine.*

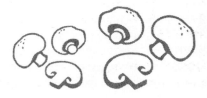

VEGETABLE RISOTTO (3)
CORE INGREDIENT
1¹/₂ cups risotto rice

FRUIT/VEGETABLES
2–3 cloves garlic, chopped
1 leek, finely sliced
1 small onion, chopped
1 small carrot
1 stick of celery
300 gm spinach

FROM THE CUPBOARD
4 T olive oil
1 L vegetable or chicken stock

HERBS AND SPICES
salt and pepper
2 T chopped parsley, basil
  and chives

1 Finely chop the carrot and
celery in a food processor
2 Heat the olive oil, add the
onion and leek and sauté for 3
to 4 mins
3 Add the garlic, carrot and
celery and continue to sauté for
another minute
4 Slowly add the stock stirring
all the time until the rice is soft
(about 20 minutes)
5 Stir in the spinach, season to
taste and continue cooking until
the spinach is just wilted
6 Just before serving stir in an
extra tablespoon of olive oil and
garnish with chopped herbs.

PREPARATION TIME:
5 minutes/COOKING TIME:
30 minutes

RISOTTO SUGGESTIONS
● Risotto with roast vegetables
● Risotto with peas, snowpeas,
asparagus and red pepper
● Risotto with zucchini
● Risotto with green beans and
red peppers

COUSCOUS WITH FRESH VEGETABLES (3)
CORE INGREDIENT
400 gm instant couscous

FRUIT/VEGETABLES
1 small onion, chopped
2–3 cloves garlic, chopped
¹/₂ cucumber, diced
10–12 cherry tomatoes, chopped
2 T lemon juice

FROM THE CUPBOARD
600 ml boiling water
4 T olive oil

HERBS AND SPICES
1 T fresh parsley
1 T fresh mint, chopped
salt and pepper to taste

1 Pour boiling water over the
couscous, and leave it to absorb
the moisture (about 5 minutes)
2 Heat the olive oil, add the
onion and stir-fry for 3 to 4

minutes, add the garlic and continue to stir-fry for another minute

3 Mix the chopped vegetables and herbs with the couscous, add the onion and garlic, any olive oil left in the pan, the extra olive oil and lemon juice

4 Stir gently to mix well, season to taste and serve.

PREPARATION TIME:
3–4 minutes/COOKING TIME:
5 minutes

COUSCOUS WITH ROCKET, CHICKEN AND PINE NUTS (6)
CORE INGREDIENT
2–3 chicken breasts, sliced

FRUIT/VEGETABLES
2–3 cloves garlic, minced
4–6 spring onions, sliced
250 gm rocket, torn into pieces
12 cherry tomatoes, halved
3 T lemon juice

FROM THE CUPBOARD
2 cups of couscous
3 cups of water
3 T olive oil
1 cup of pine nuts

HERBS AND SPICES
chopped parsley
chopped mint
salt and pepper to taste

1 Pour boiling water over the couscous, and leave it to absorb the moisture (about 5 minutes)

2 Toast, but be careful not to burn, the pine nuts

3 Heat the oil, add the garlic, and sliced chicken and stir-fry for 3 to 4 minutes until the chicken is cooked through

4 Toss the rocket, tomatoes, spring onions, pine nuts, chopped parsley, mint, chicken, any remaining olive oil and lemon juice through the couscous and season to taste. Add more olive oil if necessary.

PREPARATION TIME:
3–4 minutes/COOKING TIME:
5 minutes

COUSCOUS WITH ROCKET, BEETROOT AND WALNUTS (3)
CORE INGREDIENT
400 gm instant couscous

FRUIT/VEGETABLES
1 small red onion, chopped
300 gm cooked beetroot, chopped
125 gm rocket
2 mandarins, peeled and chopped
2 T lemon juice

FROM THE CUPBOARD
600 gm boiling water
100 gm walnuts, chopped
3 T olive oil

HERBS AND SPICES
1 T chopped chives
1 T chopped parsley
1 T ground cumin
salt and pepper to taste

1 Pour boiling water over the couscous, and leave it to absorb the moisture (about 5 minutes)
2 Heat 1 tablespoon of the oil and fry the walnuts for 2 to 3 minutes
3 Mix all the ingredients with the couscous, season to taste and serve.

PREPARATION TIME:
5–6 minutes/COOKING TIME:
5 minutes

COUSCOUS WITH TOMATO, ASPARAGUS AND PINE NUTS (3)

CORE INGREDIENT
400 gm instant couscous

FRUIT/VEGETABLES
12–16 asparagus spears
12–16 snowpeas
12–16 cherry tomatoes, cut
  in half
2 T lemon juice

FROM THE CUPBOARD
600 ml boiling water
100 gm pine nuts
3–4 T olive oil

HERBS AND SPICES
salt and pepper to taste
3 T fresh basil or parsley and
  mint leaves, coarsely shredded

1 Pour boiling water over the couscous, and leave it to absorb the moisture (about 5 minutes)
2 Heat one tablespoon of olive oil in a pan, add the pine nuts and fry gently until they turn golden brown, then tip the nuts and oil into the couscous and mix well
3 Cut the asparagus into 3 to 4 pieces, halve the snowpeas and steam or boil separately until just tender (about 2 to 3 minutes for the asparagus and 1 minute for the snowpeas). Cool them immediately under cold water and put them in the fridge to chill
4 When cool, mix with the couscous, add the halved cherry tomatoes, basil, mint, remaining olive oil and lemon juice and toss everything together.

If you prefer, this could be served warm as soon as the vegetables are cooked.

PREPARATION TIME: 5–6 minutes/COOKING TIME: 5 minutes, plus 10 minutes to cool

COUSCOUS WITH FRUIT AND VEGETABLES (3)
CORE INGREDIENT
400 gm instant couscous

FRUIT/VEGETABLES
1 cucumber
6–8 spring onions
1/3 cup of lemon juice
3 fresh peaches or nectarines, diced
green salad

FROM THE CUPBOARD
600 ml boiling water
1/3 cup of olive oil

HERBS AND SPICES
1/2 cup of fresh parsley, chopped
1/2 cup of fresh mint, chopped
salt to taste
1 T coriander, chopped

1 Pour boiling water over the couscous, and leave it to absorb the moisture (about 5 minutes)
2 Peel and finely chop the cucumber and spring onions and add to a bowl with the parsley, mint, coriander and a sprinkle of salt
3 Add the couscous to the vegetables and mix through
4 Just before serving add

peaches or nectarines and serve with mixed green salad leaves.

PREPARATION TIME: 8–10 minutes/COOKING TIME: 5 minutes

POLENTA WITH ONION AND CHILLI (3)
CORE INGREDIENT
1 1/2 cups of instant polenta

FRUIT/VEGETABLES
1 onion, chopped
2 cloves garlic, chopped

FROM THE CUPBOARD
3 cups of chicken stock
1 T olive oil

HERBS AND SPICES
1 small red chilli
salt and pepper
1 T fresh oregano

1 Sauté the onion in a little oil until the onion is brown
2 Add the garlic, chilli and oregano and sauté for another 2 mins
3 Add the stock, bring to the boil and simmer for 5 minutes
4 Add the polenta and simmer, stirring constantly, for about 15 minutes or until the mixture is thick.

PREPARATION TIME:
1–2 minutes/COOKING TIME:
25 minutes

VARIATION:
● *Serve with bean stew. Polenta goes particularly well with stews and stir fries where there is plenty of sauce. Pour into a flat baking tray and leave to cool for a couple of hours. The polenta can either be cut into slices and fried or warmed in the oven. Eat it spread with dips, roasted vegetables and/or a salad.*

7.2 MEAN BEANS

It is best to buy these dry and loose, but they need soaking overnight and then cooking for 1 to 2 hours. Occasionally when pushed for time it is all right to use canned beans.

BEAN CURD

There is nothing mysterious about bean curd (tofu). It simply derives from the soya bean which is a close relative of peas and beans, which are familiar to all of us. Unlike peas and beans soya contains the full range of proteins that we need in our diet. It has been a staple food for millions of people in Asia for over 4000 years.

Substituting bean curd (or soya generally) for animal products:
● *Reduces cholesterol and triglycerides, helping the heart and respiratory system*
● *Increases protective phytoestrogens and substances that prevent cancers forming their own blood supply*
● *Increases levels of antioxidants which remove free radicals which can damage cells*
● *Protects against osteoporosis*
● *Eliminates growth factors and hormones and reduces hormone-mimicking chemicals that are implicated in breast, prostate and other hormone-dependent cancers (endometrial, ovarian and testicular).*

FEED THE WORLD ONE ACRE OF FARMLAND WILL FEED ONE ADULT FOR:
● ***77 DAYS IF USED FOR BEEF***
● ***527 DAYS IF USED FOR WHEAT***
● ***6 YEARS IF USED FOR SOYA – SO IT IS ENVIRONMENTALLY FRIENDLY***

Bean curd has an unusual texture and some people find it tasteless, but it absorbs flavours well and quickly, it requires no lengthy cooking and it is very easily digested. People quickly acquire a taste for good bean curd so shop around in Asian and healthfood stores or supermarkets until you find the ones you prefer. We like the smooth, silken ones best.

BEAN CURD IS ALSO SOLD AS TOFU AND A FERMENTED VERSION POPULAR IN INDONESIA IS CALLED TEMPEH.

BAKED BEAN CURD (TOFU) WITH BROCCOLI AND ALMONDS (1)

CORE INGREDIENT
1 packet bean curd, cubed

FRUIT/VEGETABLES
2–3 cloves garlic, chopped
1 cup of broccoli, cut into small
  florets
1 cup of green beans or
  asparagus, cut into 3 cm lengths
1 cup of snowpeas, cut in half
4–6 spring onions, diced
1 T fresh ginger, minced

FROM THE CUPBOARD
3 T sesame oil
2 T soya sauce
1 T mirin or white wine
  vinegar or dry sherry
2 T olive, sunflower or
  peanut oil

1 T sesame seeds
1/2 cup of almond slivers

HERBS AND SPICES
2 T coriander or basil

1 Shake together 2 tablespoons of the sesame oil, soya sauce, garlic and ginger and pour over the bean curd in a baking dish. Leave to marinate for 2 hours
2 Put the tofu in a preheated 180°C oven and bake for 30 minutes, turning halfway through cooking
3 Toast the almonds and sesame seeds separately for a few minutes
4 Steam or boil all the vegetables separately until they are just tender and mix them together with the tofu in a serving bowl
5 Mix together the remaining sesame oil, olive oil, and mirin or vinegar and toss with the baked tofu and vegetables
6 Serve with steamed rice and sprinkle with chopped coriander or basil.

PREPARATION TIME:
10 minutes, plus 60 minutes to marinate/COOKING TIME:
30 minutes

BEAN CURD AND AUBERGINE WITH CHILLI (1)

CORE INGREDIENT
1 packet bean curd, cut into thin slices

FRUIT/VEGETABLES
1 small onion
3–4 cloves garlic
250 gm aubergine, diced
1 T lime or lemon juice

FROM THE CUPBOARD
2 T olive oil
1 T soya sauce

HERBS AND SPICES
1–2 red chillies
1/2 tsp salt
1 tsp black pepper
1/4 cup of coriander
1 T chopped chives
1 T chopped basil

1 Put the garlic, chilli, salt, coriander and black pepper with 1 tablespoon of the oil into a food processor and blend into a smooth paste
2 Heat the oil in a pan before adding the onion and stir-fry for 2 to 3 minutes
3 Add the spice mix and stir-fry for another 1 to 2 minutes, then add the bean curd and continue to fry until it turns golden brown then remove it and keep warm

4 Add the diced aubergine to the pan and fry until it is soft adding a little more oil as necessary
5 Stir in the bean curd, soya sauce and the lemon or lime juice and serve sprinkled with chopped chives and basil leaves.

PREPARATION TIME: 3–4 minutes/COOKING TIME: 10–15 mins

BEAN CURD AND SPINACH CURRY (4)

CORE INGREDIENT
1 packet bean curd (tofu), cubed

FRUIT/VEGETABLES
1 large red onion, chopped
1 T fresh ginger, minced
3–4 cloves garlic, chopped
3 large vine-ripened tomatoes, chopped
2 red peppers, chopped
1 orange pepper, chopped
300 gm baby spinach leaves
1 T lime or lemon juice

FROM THE CUPBOARD
2 T olive oil
1 T sesame oil
3/4 cup of coconut milk
1 tsp fish sauce
1/4 cup of chicken or vegetable stock

HERBS AND SPICES
1 red or green chilli, chopped
  (or to taste)
1 stick lemon grass, chopped
5–6 lime leaves
2 T fresh coriander

1 Heat the olive oil and stir-fry
the onion for 3 to 4 minutes
until it has turned golden brown
2 Add the garlic, ginger, chillies,
lemon grass and stir-fry for
another minute
3 Add the tomatoes, peppers,
lime leaves and bean curd and
stir gently so that it is coated
with the mixture
4 Add the coconut milk, stock
and fish sauce and simmer for 3
to 4 minutes
5 Add the spinach and sesame
oil and stir-fry until the spinach
is just wilted
6 Sprinkle with the lemon juice,
season to taste and serve
garnished with chopped
coriander.

PREPARATION TIME: 10 mins
COOKING TIME: 10–12 mins

BEAN CURD WITH BEAN SPROUTS AND COCONUT MILK (4)
CORE INGREDIENT
1 packet bean curd, cubed
8 large green prawns, cut into
  pieces (optional)

FRUIT/VEGETABLES
1 small onion, sliced
4 cloves garlic, minced
1 T ginger, minced
4 spring onions, chopped
2 tsp lemon juice
500 gm bean sprouts

FROM THE CUPBOARD
2 T olive or peanut oil
1 tsp sesame oil
1/4 cup of coconut milk

HERBS AND SPICES
1 red chilli, chopped or 1 tsp
  chilli sauce
1/2 tsp turmeric
salt to taste
2 T fresh coriander

1 Heat a wok, add the oil and
fry the mustard seeds, onions
and chilli for 2 to 3 minutes
2 Add the garlic, ginger, prawns
and turmeric and continue to
fry for about 2 to 3 minutes
until the prawns turn pink
3 Add the coconut milk and
bean curd, bring to a gentle boil
and simmer for another 2 to 3
minutes until the bean curd is
heated through
4 Add the spring onions and
bean sprouts and cook for
another minute
5 Serve with steamed rice or
rice noodles garnished with
chopped coriander.

PREPARATION TIME:
5–6 minutes/COOKING TIME:
10 minutes

BRAISED BEAN CURD WITH SNOWPEAS (3)
CORE INGREDIENT
1 packet bean curd

FRUIT/VEGETABLES
1 T garlic, minced
1 T ginger, minced
4 spring onions, cut into 2 cm
  pieces
125 gm snowpeas
1 large onion, chopped

FROM THE CUPBOARD
2 T olive oil
1 T tomato paste
1 T oyster sauce
1–2 T water

HERBS AND SPICES
2 T fresh coriander
5–6 lime leaves
1 stick lemon grass, chopped
salt and pepper to taste
1 fresh red chilli, chopped
2 tsp chilli sauce

1 Cut the bean curd into cubes
and sauté in olive oil at medium
heat until they are brown on
both sides. Put to one side
2 In the same pan, add the
chopped onions, lemon grass,
lime leaves, chilli and chilli

sauce and sauté for 2 to 3
minutes
3 Add the tomato paste, garlic
and ginger and continue to
sauté for another 1 to 2 minutes
4 Add the snowpeas, spring
onions, oyster sauce and the
fried bean curd and a little
water, cover and heat through
for 1 to 2 minutes. Serve
garnished with fresh coriander.

PREPARATION TIME: 3–4 mins
COOKING TIME: 8–10 mins

STIR-FRIED BEAN CURD WITH BEAN SPROUTS AND OYSTER SAUCE (3)
CORE INGREDIENT
1 packet bean curd

FRUIT/VEGETABLES
2–3 cloves garlic, minced
100 gm bean sprouts
4 spring onions, sliced
1 red pepper, sliced

FROM THE CUPBOARD
2 T peanut or sunflower oil
4 T oyster sauce

HERBS AND SPICES
1 red chilli, chopped
black pepper

1 Heat the oil and sauté the
garlic and chilli for about 1
minute

2 Add the bean curd, red pepper and oyster sauce and sauté for another 2 to 3 minutes
3 Add the bean sprouts and spring onions, season to taste with black pepper (you should not need any salt), sauté for another minute and serve with steamed rice.

PREPARATION TIME:
2–3 minutes/COOKING TIME:
5 minutes

STIR-FRIED BEAN CURD WITH MIXED VEGETABLES (3)

CORE INGREDIENT
1 packet bean curd, cubed

FRUIT/VEGETABLES
3–4 garlic cloves, minced
1/2 pumpkin, peeled and chopped
1/2 cup of celery, sliced
6–8 asparagus spears, cut into 5 cm lengths
125 gm baby corn
60 gm snowpeas
8–12 baby shitake mushrooms or baby mushrooms
4–6 spring onions
1 T lemon or lime juice

FROM THE CUPBOARD
2 T peanut or olive oil
1 T soya sauce
1/4 of cup of water (or mushroom water)

HERBS AND SPICES
1 red chilli, chopped
2 T fresh coriander, chopped

1 Soak the dried mushrooms in boiling water and leave them to absorb the water for about 20 minutes, drain and reserve the liquid
2 Heat the oil and fry the garlic and chilli for one minute
3 Add the pumpkin and celery and continue to sauté for 3 to 4 minutes
4 Add the asparagus, corn, mushrooms, bean curd and water, cover and simmer briskly for about 3–4 minutes until the vegetables are just cooked
5 Add the snowpeas, spring onions, fish sauce, soya sauce and lemon juice and stir gently. Continue to cook for one minute until it is all warmed through
6 Serve garnished with fresh coriander.

PREPARATION TIME:
10 minutes, plus 20 minutes for marinating/COOKING TIME:
10 minutes

STIR-FRIED BEAN CURD WITH ASPARAGUS AND GREEN BEANS (3)

CORE INGREDIENT
1 packet bean curd, sliced

FRUIT/VEGETABLES
2–3 cloves garlic, minced
1 T ginger, minced
3–4 asparagus spears per
person, cut into 5 cm lengths
125 gm green beans, cut into 5
cm pieces
8–12 dried shitake
mushrooms
4 spring onions

FROM THE CUPBOARD
2 T olive oil
1 T sesame oil
2 T soya sauce
2 T mirin
1/4 cup of mushroom water
(or water)

HERBS AND SPICES
5–6 sage leaves, torn into pieces

1 Soak the mushrooms in
boiling water for about 20
minutes, drain and reserve
the liquid
2 Heat the oil, add the garlic,
ginger, asparagus and green
beans and sauté for one minute
3 Add the mirin and mushroom
water and continue to sauté
until the asparagus and beans

are just cooked – about 3 to 4
minutes
4 Add the bean curd and sage,
season to taste and cook or 2 to
3 minutes turning the bean curd
once.

PREPARATION TIME: 5 minutes
COOKING TIME: 6–8 minutes

BEAN CURD WITH SNOWPEAS AND RED PEPPER (3)

CORE INGREDIENT
1 packet bean curd, cut into
cubes

FRUIT/VEGETABLES
1 large onion, chopped
1 tsp ginger, minced
4 cloves garlic, chopped
4 spring onions, sliced
150 gm snowpeas
1 red pepper, sliced

FROM THE CUPBOARD
1/4 cup water or vegetable stock
1 T tomato paste
1 T soya sauce
1 tsp fish sauce
2 T olive oil
1 T sesame oil

HERBS AND SPICES
2 tsp chilli sauce
1/2 cup of chopped fresh parsley

1 Heat the olive oil and fry the

bean curd over a moderate heat until it turns brown on both sides and reserve
2 Add the onions to the pan and fry for 2 to 3 minutes
3 Add the garlic, ginger, red pepper, chilli, and tomato paste and fry for 2 to 3 minutes
4 Add the snowpeas, spring onions, soya sauce, bean curd, sesame oil, fish sauce and water, cover and cook for 2 to 3 minutes
5 Serve garnished with chopped parsley.

PREPARATION TIME: 5 minutes
COOKING TIME: 6–8 minutes

TOFU SUGGESTIONS
● Grilled tofu with roasted vegetables (page 154)
● Tofu with sautéed fennel and red pepper
● Tofu with stir-fried snap peas, snowpeas and asparagus (page 157–8)

BAKED BEANS (3/4)
CORE INGREDIENT
250 gm dried cannellini beans, or 2 cans cannellini beans

FRUIT/VEGETABLES
1 large onion, chopped
3–4 cloves garlic, chopped
4–5 medium tomatoes, or 1 can Italian tomatoes, chopped

FROM THE CUPBOARD
4 T olive oil
2 T tomato paste

HERBS AND SPICES
1 bunch sage leaves, chopped
salt and freshly ground black pepper

1 Soak the beans overnight, drain and transfer to a large pot of fresh water. Bring to the boil, reduce to a low heat, cover and simmer for 2 hours, then drain. Alternatively rinse and drain the canned beans
2 Heat the olive oil, add the onion and cook for 3 to 4 minutes, then add the garlic and continue to stir-fry for 1 to 2 minutes
3 Add the tomatoes, reduce the heat and simmer for 30 minutes until the juice begins to reduce
4 Add the beans and sage to the tomato sauce and season to taste. Add a little water if necessary, heat through and serve.

PREPARATION TIME: 5 mins, plus overnight soaking if using dried beans/COOKING TIME: 30–35 mins, plus 2 hours if using dried beans

BAKED BEANS ON TOAST PROVIDE A FULL RANGE OF ESSENTIAL PROTEINS.

BEAN AND TUNA SALAD (6)
CORE INGREDIENT
1 fillet of fresh tuna

FRUIT/VEGETABLES
1 small red onion, chopped
2 sticks celery, chopped
2 vine-ripened tomatoes,
  chopped
1 green pepper, chopped

FROM THE CUPBOARD
1 can cannellini or borlotti
  beans
1 can red kidney beans
1/4 cup of olive oil
2 T red wine vinegar

HERBS AND SPICES
1 tsp salt
2 T chopped parsley
black pepper

1 Cut the tuna into small cubes. Sear in a griddle pan for 1 to 2 minutes each side, until it has changed colour on the outside but is still pink on the inside
2 Drain and rinse the beans and put them into a salad bowl, add the tuna, chopped tomatoes, celery and green pepper,
sprinkle with salt and mix together gently
3 Mix together the olive oil, red wine vinegar and black pepper, pour over the bean salad and serve immediately sprinkled with chopped parsley.

PREPARATION TIME:
10 minutes/COOKING TIME:
3–4 minutes

SHORT CUT: This can be made with a can of good Italian tuna packed in olive oil.

CANNELLINI BEAN SALAD (3)
CORE INGREDIENT
125 gm dried cannellini beans
  (or 1 can cannellini beans)

FRUIT/VEGETABLES
1 large onion
2–3 cloves garlic
4–5 medium tomatoes

FROM THE CUPBOARD
4 T olive oil

HERBS AND SPICES
3 T mixed Italian herbs such as
  parsley, oregano and sage
1 T chopped chives
salt and pepper

1 Soak the dried beans overnight, drain and cook in

plenty of water for about 2 hours or drain, rinse and heat a can of beans

2 Process the onion, garlic, tomatoes, olive oil and herbs in a food processor until coarsely chopped

3 Mix together the warm beans and the tomato mixture, add lots of black pepper and season to taste

4 Serve warm or at room temperature (do not chill in the fridge).

PREPARATION TIME: 5 minutes/COOKING TIME: 5 minutes, plus 2 hours if using dried beans

CANNELLINI BEAN, LAMB AND VEGETABLE STEW (7)
CORE INGREDIENT
350 gm leg of lamb, cubed

FRUIT/VEGETABLES
3–4 cloves garlic, minced
10–12 small shallots, peeled
2–3 carrots, sliced
3–4 red potatoes, cubed
1 sweet potato, cubed
1–2 parsnips, cubed
1 cup of peas
1 cup of corn

FROM THE CUPBOARD
3 T olive oil
1 can cannellini beans

1 L vegetable stock
1/2 cup of pearl barley

HERBS AND SPICES
1 sprig rosemary
2 sprigs thyme
2 bay leaves
salt and pepper
2 T parsley

1 Heat the olive oil and brown the lamb

2 Add the garlic, rosemary, thyme, bay leaves and stock and simmer slowly for about 20 minutes

3 Add the shallots, carrots, potatoes, parsnips, sweet potato and barley and simmer for another 30 to 40 minutes

4 Add the peas, corn and tinned beans, heat through and season to taste

5 Serve in soup bowls garnished with parsley.

PREPARATION TIME: 10 minutes/COOKING TIME: 60 minutes

CHICKPEA CURRY (3)
CORE INGREDIENT
1 can chickpeas

FRUIT/VEGETABLES
2 medium onions, chopped
3–4 cloves garlic, chopped
3–4 tomatoes, chopped

1 T ginger, minced
2 T lemon juice

FROM THE CUPBOARD
1/2 cup olive oil
1/2 cup water

HERBS AND SPICES
1 tsp ground cumin
1 tsp ground coriander
1 tsp cayenne pepper
2 green chillies
2 T fresh coriander

1 Heat the oil and fry the onions until they turn golden brown, about 4 to 5 minutes
2 Add all the other spices except the fresh coriander and continue to stir-fry for another 1 to 2 minutes
3 Add the chickpeas and tomatoes and simmer for about 20 minutes
4 Stir in the lemon juice and fresh coriander
5 Serve with steamed rice and/or another curry.

PREPARATION TIME:
3–4 minutes/COOKING TIME:
25–30 mins

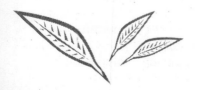

CHICKPEAS WITH PUMPKIN AND SWEET POTATO (3)

CORE INGREDIENT
125 gm dried chickpeas
  or 1 can chickpeas

FRUIT/VEGETABLES
1 small pumpkin, chopped
1 sweet potato, chopped
1 carrot, chopped
2 small zucchini, sliced
1 onion, chopped
3 tomatoes, chopped
3 cloves garlic, minced
1 T ginger, minced

FROM THE CUPBOARD
3 T olive oil
2 T raisins
2 T pine nuts
3 cups vegetable stock

HERBS AND SPICES
1 tsp cumin
1 tsp paprika
1/2 tsp turmeric
1 tsp cayenne pepper
1 tsp salt
1 cinnamon stick
2 star anise
1 T coriander
1 T parsley
1 T mint

1 Soak the beans overnight, rinse and cook for 2 hours, or drain and rinse the canned beans

2 Toast the pine nuts in a shallow pan until they change colour

3 Heat the oil and sauté the onion, cinnamon stick and anise for 2 to 3 minutes then add the garlic, ginger, cumin, paprika, turmeric, cayenne pepper and salt and continue to sauté for another minute

4 Add the tomatoes and continue to fry for another 2 to 3 minutes

5 Add the chickpeas, pumpkin, sweet potato, carrot, zucchini, raisins and stock, bring to boil, reduce to a slow simmer, cover and cook for about 15 to 20 minutes

6 Stir through the chopped herbs and serve with wild rice or couscous.

PREPARATION TIME: 10–15 minutes/COOKING TIME: 25–30 mins

CHICKPEAS WITH SPINACH (3)
CORE INGREDIENT
1 can chickpeas (or dried equivalent)

FRUIT/VEGETABLES
2 onions, chopped
4–5 cloves garlic, chopped
450 gm spinach
2 T lemon juice

FROM THE CUPBOARD
4 T olive oil

HERBS AND SPICES
1 T ground cumin
1 tsp cayenne
1 tsp black pepper
salt to taste

1 Heat the olive oil and sauté the onions for 2 to 3 minutes

2 Add the minced garlic, cayenne and cumin and sauté for another minute

3 Add the chickpeas and just enough water to cover them and the lemon juice and simmer for about 30 minutes

4 Add the spinach, lemon juice, pepper and salt and continue to cook until the spinach has just wilted.

PREPARATION TIME: 3 minutes/COOKING TIME: 30–40 mins

CHILLI BEANS (4)
CORE INGREDIENT
2 cans red kidney beans

FRUIT/VEGETABLES
1 onion, chopped
3–4 cloves garlic, chopped
3–4 vine-ripened tomatoes, chopped
1 red pepper, chopped
1 cup of frozen corn

FROM THE CUPBOARD
1 T olive oil
1/4 cup of vegetable stock or
   water

HERBS AND SPICES
1 T cumin
2 tsp coriander
1 tsp cayenne pepper
   (or to taste)
2 T fresh coriander

1 Heat the oil in a saucepan,
add the onion and fry for 2 to 3
minutes, add the garlic, cumin,
coriander and cayenne pepper
and stir-fry for another 1 to 2
minutes
2 Add the kidney beans, pepper,
tomatoes and stock, stir well and
bring to a boil, then reduce the
heat and simmer uncovered for
15 to 20 minutes. Add a little
more water if necessary
3 Add the corn and heat
through
4 Serve on toast garnished with
fresh coriander.

PREPARATION TIME:
8–10 minutes/COOKING TIME:
25–30 mins

**CURRIED LENTILS WITH
VEGETABLES (3)**
CORE INGREDIENT
1 1/2 cups of red lentils

FRUIT/VEGETABLES
150 gm broccoli, cut into florets
100 gm cauliflower, cut into
   florets
1 onion, chopped
3–4 cloves garlic, minced
2 potatoes, scrubbed and cut
   into cubes
2 carrots, sliced

FROM THE CUPBOARD
2 T olive oil
1 L vegetable stock

HERBS AND SPICES
1 tsp garam masala
1 tsp ground cumin
1 tsp ground coriander
1 tsp cayenne pepper
2 T chopped coriander
   or parsley
salt and pepper to taste

1 Rinse and drain the lentils
2 Heat the oil and sauté the
onion for 2 to 3 minutes then
add the garlic and all the spices
except the fresh coriander or
parsley and fry for another
minute
3 Add the potatoes, carrot, lentils
and the stock, season to taste and
simmer for about 10 minutes
4 Add the broccoli and
cauliflower and continue to
simmer until the vegetables are
tender, about another 10 to 15
minutes.

5 Serve with steamed rice or noodles, garnished with chopped coriander or parsley.

PREPARATION TIME:
10 minutes/COOKING TIME:
30 minutes

DHAL (SPICY LENTILS) (3)
CORE INGREDIENT
1 cup of green lentils

FRUIT/VEGETABLES
1 cooking apple, peeled, cored
  and chopped
1 medium onion (optional)

FROM THE CUPBOARD
2 T olive oil
2-3 cups of water

HERBS AND SPICES
1 tsp turmeric
1 tsp salt
1 tsp cayenne pepper
  (or to taste)
2 bay leaves

1 Heat the oil and fry the lentils (and onions) for 2 mins, stirring
2 Add the spices and fry briefly
3 Add two cups of water, cover the pan and simmer gently
4 Add the chopped apple after about 20 minutes and continue to simmer until the lentils are soft (about another 10 minutes). If the lentils become dry before

they are cooked just add more water to the pan.
5 Serve with steamed rice and other curries.

PREPARATION TIME:
1-2 minutes/COOKING TIME:
30 minutes

LENTIL, BEAN SPROUT AND RICE SALAD (3)
CORE INGREDIENT
1 cup of brown or green lentils

FRUIT/VEGETABLES
1-2 cloves garlic, chopped
1½ cups of fresh mung beans
  or bean sprouts
1 small red onion, chopped

FROM THE CUPBOARD
4 T olive oil
2 T balsamic vinegar
1 cup of long grain brown rice
2 cups of water

HERBS AND SPICES
1 tsp cumin powder
salt and pepper to taste
2 T fresh mint leaves
2 T fresh chopped parsley

1 Cook the rice in two cups of water, seasoned to taste and put in the fridge to cool
2 Heat one tablespoon of oil, add the garlic, cumin and lentils and stir-fry for 1 minute. Add

the water and simmer for 30 to 40 minutes until the lentils are soft. Add more water if necessary

3 Mix together all the ingredients, except the mint and parsley, then put the salad in the fridge to cool

4 Mix in the herbs just before serving.

PREPARATION TIME:
2–3 mins/COOKING TIME:
30 mins, plus time to cool

LENTILS AND RICE WITH CARAMELISED ONIONS (3)
CORE INGREDIENT
1 cup of basmati rice

FRUIT/VEGETABLES
2 medium onions, chopped
3–4 cloves garlic, minced
1 cucumber, chopped
2–3 tomatoes, chopped
4 spring onions, chopped

FROM THE CUPBOARD
5 T olive oil
1 cup brown or green lentils
4 cups water or vegetable stock

HERBS AND SPICES
1 T cumin
salt and pepper to taste
chopped herbs – parsley or basil or chives or coriander

1 Caramelise the onions by sautéing gently in 3 tablespoons of olive oil until the onions become very dark brown, drain and set aside

2 Heat one tablespoon of oil and sauté the garlic for one minute, add the lentils, rice and cumin and sauté for another minute

3 Add the stock, cover and simmer for about 45 minutes until the rice and lentils are cooked

4 Allow to cool slightly then mix through the cucumber, tomato, spring onions and chopped herbs and season to taste

5 Serve with the caramelised onions.

PREPARATION TIME:
10 minutes/COOKING TIME:
45–50 mins

RED LENTIL SALAD (3)
CORE INGREDIENT
1 1/2 cups red lentils

FRUIT/VEGETABLES
4 cloves garlic, minced
1 T ginger, minced
150 gm mixed salad leaves
1 chicory, sliced
1 T lime juice

FROM THE CUPBOARD
2 T olive oil
3 cups vegetable or chicken
stock

HERBS AND SPICES
1 red chilli, chopped
1 T cumin
2 T chopped mint
2 T chopped parsley
salt and pepper

1 Heat the oil and fry the garlic,
ginger, chilli and cumin for one
minute, then add the lentils and
continue to fry for another
minute
2 Add the stock and simmer
until the lentils are soft and the
liquid has been absorbed (about
20 to 30 minutes)
3 Stir through the lime juice,
mint, parsley and salt and pepper
to taste
4 Serve with mixed salad leaves
and chicory.

PREPARATION TIME:
2–3 minutes/COOKING TIME:
20–30 mins

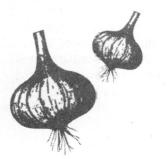

7.3 VITAL VEGETABLES

Vegetables are crucial for good
health and are a particularly
important part of the Plant
Programme. Unfortunately,
many people do not enjoy
vegetables, or else eat them
covered with 'gloppy' dairy-
based sauces. Here are some
healthy and much more exciting
vegetable dishes for you to try.

BAKED POTATOES – BAKE
THEM IN THE OVEN
THE OLD-FASHIONED WAY –
NOT IN A MICROWAVE.
THEY ARE DELICIOUS
SERVED WITH A SALAD
OR ON THEIR OWN
ACCOMPANIED BY ANY
OF THE DELICIOUS DIPS
DESCRIBED IN THE
'MEALS ON THE RUN'
SECTION.

SOME IDEAS FOR
FILLINGS OR GARNISHES
FOR BAKED POTATOES
INCLUDE:
● Basil or parsley pesto
● Chopped fresh herbs
with olive oil
● Cucumber and soya
yoghurt dip
● Guacamole

- Hummus
- Pineapple and corn salsa
- Sautéed mushrooms
- Tomato and onion salsa

CAULIFLOWER AND POTATO CURRY (3)
CORE INGREDIENT
1 small cauliflower, cut into
  florets

FRUIT/VEGETABLES
1 large onion, coarsely chopped
3 medium potatoes, scrubbed
  and diced
4 cloves garlic, chopped
1 T ginger, minced
2 large tomatoes, sliced

FROM THE CUPBOARD
1 cup of water
3 T sunflower or peanut oil

HERBS AND SPICES
1 tsp cayenne powder
1 tsp cumin powder
1 tsp garam masala
1 tsp turmeric
2 T fresh coriander leaves

1 Heat the oil in a wok and stir-
fry the onion for 2 to 3 minutes
2 Add the garlic and ginger and
fry for 1 to 2 minutes, then add
the dry spices and fry for
another 1 to 2 minutes
3 Add the cauliflower and
potato and stir for a few minutes

to coat them with the spices
4 Add the water, cover the pan
and simmer briskly for 10
minutes
5 Add the tomatoes and
continue to simmer for another
5 minutes or until all the
vegetables are tender. Sprinkle
with fresh chopped coriander
leaves.
6 Serve with plain steamed rice
or naan or with another curry
such as Dhal on page 147.

PREPARATION TIME:
10 minutes/COOKING TIME:
20–25 minutes

CAULIFLOWER WITH TAHINI AND AVOCADO SAUCE (3)
This is an interesting alternative
to cauliflower cheese.

CORE INGREDIENT
1 medium cauliflower, cut
  into florets

FRUIT/VEGETABLES
2 avocados, peeled and chopped
2–3 cloves garlic
1/2 cup of lemon juice

FROM THE CUPBOARD
1 cup of tahini paste
1/2 cup of pine nuts
1/4 cup of water
1/4 cup of olive oil

HERBS AND SPICES
1/2 tsp salt
pepper to taste
chopped parsley

1 Steam or boil the cauliflower until it is tender
2 In a food processor blend the garlic, salt, lemon juice, olive oil, tahini, avocado and water to a smooth paste
3 Roast the pine nuts in the oven until they change colour
4 Gently heat the avocado sauce in a saucepan until it is warmed through. Pour it over the cooked cauliflower and garnish it with chopped parsley and roasted pine nuts.

PREPARATION TIME:
8–10 minutes/COOKING TIME:
12–15 minutes

CURRIED CAULIFLOWER (3)
CORE INGREDIENT
1 small cauliflower, cut into florets

FRUIT/VEGETABLES
1 small onion, chopped
1 T fresh ginger, minced
3–4 cloves garlic, chopped
1 large tomato, chopped

FROM THE CUPBOARD
1/2 cup of water
2 T olive oil

HERBS AND SPICES
1/2 tsp turmeric
1/2 tsp cumin powder
1/2 tsp cayenne pepper
1/2 tsp mustard seeds
1/2 tsp cumin seeds
1/2 tsp fennel seeds
salt and pepper to taste
1 T chopped coriander

1 Heat the olive oil briefly in a wok and add the mustard, fennel and cumin seeds and fry for about 1 minute.
2 Add the onion and fry for another 2 to 3 minutes, then add the garlic, ginger and ground spices and continue to fry for another minute
3 Add the cauliflower and stir-fry for 2 to 3 minutes. Add the water and chopped tomato, cover and cook for approximately 15 minutes until the cauliflower is tender.
4 Serve with chopped coriander and rice or with another curry. This is good reheated.

PREPARATION TIME:
5 minutes/COOKING TIME:
20–25 minutes

VARIATIONS:
● *Add green or red chillies.*
● *Add chopped green or red pepper or fennel.*

GREEN BEANS WITH GARLIC (3)
CORE INGREDIENT
450 gm green beans

FRUIT/VEGETABLES
2–3 cloves garlic, chopped
1 T lemon juice

FROM THE CUPBOARD
2 T olive oil
1 T pine nuts or almonds

HERBS AND SPICES
salt to taste

1 Steam the green beans for approximately 8 minutes (this leaves them still a little crunchy)
2 Toast the pine nuts or almonds until they change colour
3 Heat the olive oil, add the garlic and stir-fry for 1 minute, then add the beans and sauté for 2 to 3 minutes
4 Serve sprinkled with the lemon juice and a little coarsely ground sea salt.

PREPARATION TIME:
3–4 minutes/COOKING TIME:
10 minutes

VARIATION:
● *This dish can be served cold. Simply rinse the steamed beans* under cold water, before tossing with the other ingredients. Season to taste and leave to cool (do not refrigerate).
● *Use zucchini.*

SAUTÉED AUBERGINES
CORE INGREDIENT
2 aubergines, cut into 1 cm-thick slices

FRUIT/VEGETABLES
2–3 cloves garlic, minced

FROM THE CUPBOARD
4 T olive oil

HERBS AND SPICES
salt and pepper
2 T fresh basil

1 Heat the oil in a frying pan and sauté the garlic for one minute
2 Add the aubergine, season to taste and stir to ensure it is well coated with the olive oil
3 Sauté, turning occasionally for 6 to 8 minutes until the aubergine is soft (it will absorb the oil quickly but will become 'oily' again as it continues to cook. Don't add more oil)
4 Serve sprinkled with basil.

PREPARATION TIME:
2–3 minutes/COOKING TIME:
8–10 minutes

SPICY OKRA ((3)
CORE INGREDIENT
450 gm okra, topped and tailed
  and halved

FRUIT/VEGETABLES
1 tomato, chopped
2 medium onions, sliced
3–4 cloves garlic, minced
2 T fresh lemon juice

FROM THE CUPBOARD
1/4 cup olive oil

HERBS AND SPICES
2–3 green chillies, chopped
3–4 curry leaves or 2 bay leaves
1 tsp salt
2 T chopped coriander leaves

1 Heat the oil and fry the
onions for 2 to 3 minutes.
Add the garlic and chilli and
continue to fry for 1 to 2
minutes
2 Gradually add the okra,
mixing gently so as not to break
the pieces, and stir-fry for about
3 to 4 minutes.
3 Add the chopped tomato,
season to taste and continue
frying for another 5 minutes.
4 Pour over the lemon juice,
sprinkle with coriander and
serve.

This is great reheated.

PREPARATION TIME:
10 minutes/COOKING TIME:
15 minutes

POTATO AND SPINACH CURRY (3)
CORE INGREDIENT
3–4 large potatoes

FRUIT/VEGETABLES
2 large onions, finely chopped
6 cloves garlic, minced
500 gm fresh spinach
4–5 Italian tomatoes, chopped

FROM THE CUPBOARD
3 T olive oil

HERBS AND SPICES
1 T ground cumin
1/2 T ground coriander
1 tsp cayenne pepper
1 tsp salt
2 cups fresh coriander

1 Boil the potatoes until they
are soft, drain and chop coarsely
2 Heat the oil and stir-fry the
onions for 3 to 4 minutes until
they become light brown. Add
the garlic and continue frying
for another minute
3 Add the salt, ground
coriander, cumin and cayenne
pepper and fry for another
minute, then add the potatoes
4 Chop the tomatoes in the
processor, add to the potatoes

and simmer, covered, for about 5 to 6 minutes.

5 Put the spinach and one cup of coriander in a food processor and chop finely. Add to the potatoes and simmer until heated through

6 Serve, sprinkled with the extra chopped fresh coriander leaves.

PREPARATION TIME:
8–10 minutes/COOKING TIME:
25–30 minutes

ROAST VEGETABLES (3)
CORE INGREDIENT
2 aubergines, cut into cubes

FRUIT/VEGETABLES
6–8 garlic cloves, chopped
250 gm cherry tomatoes
3 zucchini, cut into thick slices
2 fennel bulbs, cut into wedges
2 small red onions, cut into
  wedges
1 red pepper, cut into pieces
1 orange pepper, cut into pieces

FROM THE CUPBOARD
1/4 cup olive oil

HERBS AND SPICES
2–3 T fresh basil, parsley or coriander

1 Put all the vegetables in a large baking dish, drizzle over the olive oil and stir well to ensure all the vegetable pieces are well coated in oil. Sprinkle with plenty of fresh basil leaves

2 Roast at 180°C for 30 to 40 minutes, checking frequently after about 30 minutes to make sure they do not burn.

PREPARATION TIME:
15 minutes/COOKING TIME:
30–45 mins

VARIATIONS:
● *Use lots of whole peeled garlic cloves.*
● *Add sweet potato and/or pumpkin.*
● *Left-over roast vegetables can be made into a delicious omelette for breakfast – see instructions below.*

1 Heat the vegetables
2 Lightly beat four eggs and pour over the vegetables and either bake in the oven until the eggs have set or cook as a normal omelette finishing off the top under the grill.

SPICY CUMIN POTATOES (3)
CORE INGREDIENT
500 gm potatoes, scrubbed

FRUIT/VEGETABLES
3–4 cloves garlic, chopped

FROM THE CUPBOARD
2–3 T sunflower or peanut oil

HERBS AND SPICES
1 tsp cumin powder
1 tsp cayenne pepper

1 Boil or steam the potatoes
until they are just cooked, then
drain, cool slightly and cut them
into cubes
2 Heat the oil in a wok, add the
garlic, potatoes and spices and
stir-fry until the potatoes are
brown and crispy

PREPARATION TIME:
1–2 minutes/COOKING TIME:
30–35 mins

FRIED FENNEL POTATOES (3)
CORE INGREDIENT
500 gm potatoes, scrubbed

FRUIT/VEGETABLES
3–4 cloves garlic, sliced
2 small fennel bulbs, sliced
1 small onion, chopped

FROM THE CUPBOARD
2–3 T sunflower or peanut oil

HERBS AND SPICES
1 tsp cumin powder
1 tsp cayenne pepper

1 Boil or steam the potatoes
until they are just cooked, drain,
cool slightly and cut into cubes
2 Pour boiling water over the
fennel and leave it to blanch for
about 5 minutes then drain
3 Heat the oil, add the onion
and sauté for 3 to 4 minutes
then add the garlic, potato and
fennel and continue sautéing
until the potatoes and onions
are crisp.

PREPARATION TIME:
2–3 minutes/COOKING TIME:
30–40 mins

POTATO DISH SUGGESTIONS
● Add marinated artichokes to
boiled or steamed new potatoes,
garnished with parsley
● Serve steamed new potatoes
with stir-fried onion, garlic,
cherry tomatoes, spinach and
pine nuts.

TO MAKE MASHED
POTATO, USE OLIVE
OIL INSTEAD
OF BUTTER, ADD
CHOPPED GARLIC,
PARSLEY, SALT AND
PEPPER TO TASTE.
FOR A MILDER
TASTE USE ROAST
GARLIC.

STIR-FRIED VEGETABLES

Stir-fried vegetables are a staple dish in Asia and can be made with any mix of vegetables depending on what you have in the fridge or garden. All you have to do is add those vegetables which take longer to cook first. Alternatively, steam them before adding them to the wok, and stir-fry with the other vegetables. We have given suggested times, but these vary. Practice makes perfect. These are the sort of dishes that never taste the same twice – which make them even more interesting.

Here is a selection of combinations we like, but experiment with your favourite vegetables.

STIR-FRIED BOK CHOY AND FENNEL
CORE INGREDIENT
3–4 small bok choy, halved

FRUIT/VEGETABLES
2–3 cloves garlic, minced
1 medium fennel bulb, thinly
 sliced

FROM THE CUPBOARD
1 T olive oil
1 T soya sauce
2 tsp sesame oil
1 T water

HERBS AND SPICES
pepper

1 Heat the olive oil, add the garlic and fennel and stir-fry for 2 to 3 minutes
2 Add the bok choy, soya sauce, sesame oil and water and cover and cook for 1 to 2 minutes until the bok choy is just tender
3 Serve with steamed rice, or as an accompaniment to another dish.

PREPARATION TIME:
3–4 minutes/COOKING TIME:
5–6 minutes

STIR-FRIED SESAME AND GINGER CABBAGE
CORE INGREDIENT
1 250 gm cabbage, shredded

FRUIT/VEGETABLES
1/2 onion, thinly sliced
1 T fresh ginger, chopped
3–4 cloves garlic, finely chopped

FROM THE CUPBOARD
1 T olive oil
2 tsp sesame oil
3 T sesame seeds
1/4 cup of water

HERBS AND SPICES
salt and pepper to taste
1 red chilli, chopped (optional)

1 Toast the sesame seeds in a frying pan for 1 to 2 minutes until they start to change colour, and set aside
2 Heat the olive oil and sauté the onion for 2 to 3 minutes
3 Add the garlic, ginger and chilli and continue to sauté for another minute
4 Add the cabbage and sesame oil and stir-fry for one minute
5 Add the water and cook for 3 to 4 minutes or until just cooked
6 Serve sprinkled with sesame seeds.

PREPARATION TIME:
5 minutes/COOKING TIME:
8–10 minutes

STIR-FRIED CAULIFLOWER, ZUCCHINI AND FENNEL (3)
CORE INGREDIENT
1 small cauliflower, cut into florets

FRUIT/VEGETABLES
1 small leek, chopped
3–4 garlic cloves, minced
100 gm green beans
1 medium zucchini, sliced
2 medium tomatoes, sliced
1/2 medium fennel, sliced
1 cup of peas

FROM THE CUPBOARD
2 T olive oil
2 T light soya sauce

1 tsp sesame oil
1/2 cup of water

HERBS AND SPICES
2 T chopped coriander
1 tsp chilli sauce
salt and pepper to taste

1 Heat the oil, add the leek, garlic, cauliflower and beans and stir-fry for a few minutes
2 Add the water, cover and simmer for 5 to 7 minutes
3 Add the tomatoes, fennel and zucchini and continue to simmer for about 5 minutes, then add the frozen peas, soya sauce, chilli sauce, sesame oil, season to taste and simmer for 1 to 2 minutes until heated through
4 Serve garnished with coriander.

PREPARATION TIME:
10 minutes/COOKING TIME:
15 minutes

VARIATIONS:
● *Add mushrooms.*
● *Add green prawns or tofu when adding the tomatoes.*

STIR-FRIED ASPARAGUS, SNAP PEAS AND SNOWPEAS WITH ALMONDS (3)
CORE INGREDIENT
120 gm asparagus

FRUIT/VEGETABLES
1 T ginger, slivered
100 gm snowpeas
100 gm snap peas
1 red pepper, sliced
60 gm bean sprouts
2 spring onions, chopped

FROM THE CUPBOARD
2 T almonds
1 T olive oil
1 T mirin
1 T water

HERBS AND SPICES
2 T coriander chopped

1 Toast the almonds in the oven or in a dry pan for 2 to 3 minutes
2 Blanch the snap peas in boiling water for about 5 minutes then drain
3 Heat the olive oil, add the ginger, asparagus, red pepper and snap peas and sauté for 2 to 3 minutes
4 Add the mirin, water and snowpeas, cover and cook for 2 minutes
5 Add the bean sprouts and spring onions, sauté for one minute, and serve with the chopped coriander.

PREPARATION TIME:
5–6 minutes/COOKING TIME:
5–6 minutes

STIR-FRIED ASIAN VEGETABLES (3)
CORE INGREDIENT
1 bunch kai lan or any chinese greens, cut into thirds

FRUIT/VEGETABLES
2–3 cloves garlic, minced
4 spring onions, chopped
1 bok choy, halved
180 gm spinach
8–12 small mushrooms
60 gm snowpeas
1 cup of bean sprouts

FROM THE CUPBOARD
2 T olive oil
1 T sesame oil
2 T light soya sauce
1/2 cup of water

HERBS AND SPICES
salt to taste

1 Heat the olive oil, add the garlic and stir-fry for 1 minute
2 Add the kai lan, bok choy and mushrooms and stir-fry for 1 to 2 mins, then add the water, cover and simmer for 2 to 3 minutes
3 Add the rest of the ingredients and heat through for 1 to 2 mins.

PREPARATION TIME:
5 minutes/COOKING TIME:
5–8 minutes

STIR-FRIED SUGGESTIONS
- Mushrooms with snowpeas and pine nuts
- Sweet potato and broccoli
- Fennel, red pepper and spinach
- Asparagus, baby corn and red pepper

VEGETABLE KEBABS WITH TAHINI (3)
FRUIT/VEGETABLES
1 eggplant, cubed
4 shallots, halved
3 zucchini, thickly sliced
1 red pepper, coarsely chopped
16 cherry tomatoes
2 cloves garlic, crushed
2 T lemon juice

FROM THE CUPBOARD
1/4 cup of olive oil
1/4 cup of white wine vinegar
1/2 cup of tahini paste
1/4 cup of cold water

HERBS AND SPICES
2 T chopped parsley
1 small red chilli, chopped
1 tsp salt

1 Sprinkle the eggplant with salt and set it aside for about 30 minutes, then rinse under cold water, drain and pat dry with kitchen paper
2 Combine the olive oil, vinegar, garlic, chilli and lemon juice

3 Put the vegetables in a large dish, pour over the dressing and leave to marinate for at least an hour
4 Reserving the marinade, thread the vegetables on skewers and barbecue or grill for 3 to 4 minutes each side
5 Mix the tahini with the vegetable marinade and whisk until smooth, put in a saucepan and warm gently, pour over the kebabs and serve sprinkled with parsley.

PREPARATION TIME:
15 minutes, plus 1 hour marinating/ COOKING TIME:
6–8 minutes

VEGETABLE KEBABS WITH TOFU (3)
CORE INGREDIENT
1 packet firm bean curd (tofu)

FRUIT/VEGETABLES
1 green pepper, coarsely chopped
1 red, orange or yellow pepper, coarsely chopped
2 red onions, cut into wedges
12 small/medium mushrooms
8 cherry tomatoes

FROM THE CUPBOARD
4 T soya sauce
2 T sesame oil

HERBS AND SPICES
salt to taste

1 Cut the bean curd into 2 1/2 cm cubes and marinate in the soy sauce and sesame oil for at least 30 minutes
2 Put sequences of onion, tomato, bean curd, mushroom and capsicum on each skewer
3 Mix together the soya and sesame oils, pour over the kebabs and barbecue or grill them for about 2 to 3 minutes on each side.

PREPARATION TIME:
15–20 minutes/COOKING
TIME: 5–6 mins

The kebabs are also delicious served with the tahini sauce from the previous recipe or with Thai chilli dipping sauce.

STUFFED AUBERGINES (3)
CORE INGREDIENT
2 large aubergines

FRUIT/VEGETABLES
1 red onion, chopped
3–4 cloves garlic, minced
4–5 large tomatoes, chopped
8–10 baby mushrooms, halved

FROM THE CUPBOARD
2 T olive oil
2 T pine nuts

HERBS AND SPICES
salt and pepper to taste
2 T chopped parsley

1 Cut the aubergines in half and scoop out the flesh with a grapefruit knife without piercing the outer skin and chop finely
2 Put the skins on a baking tray, brush with olive oil and bake in a preheated 180°C oven for 20 to 30 minutes
3 Toast the pine nuts in the oven or in a dry pan for 2 to 3 minutes until they just change colour
4 In a frying pan or wok, heat the oil, add the onion and stir-fry for 2 to 3 minutes, then add the garlic, tomatoes, aubergine flesh and mushrooms, season to taste and stir-fry for 5 to 6 minutes until the vegetables are cooked
5 Spoon the vegetable mixture into the aubergine skins and serve sprinkled with plenty of parsley.

PREPARATION TIME:
10 minutes/COOKING TIME:
30 minutes

**MASHED POTATOES
WITH VEGETABLES (3)**
This recipe was contributed by Julian Lowe.

CORE INGREDIENT
3-4 medium to large potatoes

FRUIT/VEGETABLES
1 onion, finely chopped
3-4 cloves garlic, crushed
2 cups of fresh spinach
1/2 cup of frozen peas
1/2 cup of frozen corn
1/2 red pepper, chopped

FROM THE CUPBOARD
1-2 T olive oil
3 T soya milk
1 T soya spread

HERBS AND SPICES
salt and pepper to taste
parsley or coriander

1 Steam or boil the potatoes
until they are cooked. Mash the
potatoes with the soya milk and
soya spread and season to taste
2 Gently heat the olive oil in a
large frying pan, add the onions
and sauté for 2 to 3 minutes.
Add garlic and red pepper and
sauté for further 2 minutes
3 Add the peas and corn and
warm through. Then add the
spinach and herbs and cook just
until the spinach starts to wilt
4 Add the vegetables to the
potatoes and mix. Season to
taste.

PREPARATION TIME:
3-4 minutes/COOKING TIME:
20-25 mins

VARIATIONS:
● *Make leftovers into burgers and*
shallow fry them in some fresh
olive oil until they are golden
brown.
● *Serve for breakfast with a slice*
of bacon or a grilled mushroom.

VEGETABLES IN COCONUT MILK (4)
CORE INGREDIENT
600 gm mixed firm vegetables,
chopped (potatoes, pumpkin,
green beans, carrots, broccoli,
cauliflower)

FRUIT/VEGETABLES
1 large onion, finely chopped
3-4 cloves garlic, chopped
1 T ginger, minced
1 large tomato, chopped
1 T lemon juice

FROM THE CUPBOARD
2 T olive or peanut oil
1 cup of coconut milk
2 cups of vegetable stock
3 tsp coarse peanut butter

HERBS AND SPICES
1 red chilli, chopped
1 piece lemon grass, finely
   chopped
salt and pepper

1 Heat the oil in a wok, add the onion and fry it for 2 to 3 minutes

2 Add the garlic, ginger, lemon grass and chilli and continue to fry for another 1 to 2 minutes

3 Add the coconut milk and stir well then slowly add the stock stirring continuously

4 Add the vegetables and cook until they are just tender

5 Stir in the peanut butter, lemon juice and season to taste.

PREPARATION TIME:
15 minutes/COOKING TIME:
15–20 minutes

SPINACH IN OYSTER SAUCE (3)
CORE INGREDIENT
400 gm spinach

FRUIT/VEGETABLES
2–3 cloves garlic, minced

FROM THE CUPBOARD
2 T olive oil
2 T oyster sauce

HERBS AND SPICES
1 tsp chilli sauce

1 Heat the oil, add the garlic and chilli and stir-fry for 1 minute

2 Wash and drain the spinach, add to the pan with the oyster

sauce and cook for about 2 minutes until the spinach starts to wilt.

PREPARATION TIME:
1 minute/COOKING TIME:
2 minutes

VARIATION:
● *Use asparagus, bok choy or chinese greens*

VEGETABLE TEMPURA (5)
CORE INGREDIENT
1 egg

FRUIT/VEGETABLES
selection of sliced vegetables:
  onion
  sweet potato
  carrot, sliced vertically
  zucchini, sliced vertically
  aubergine

FROM THE CUPBOARD
2 cups rice flour
1/2 cups cold water
sunflower or peanut oil for
  frying

HERBS AND SPICES
chilli dipping sauce

1 Mix the flour and water to a thin consistency

2 Lightly beat the egg and whisk it into the flour

3 Dip the vegetables into the

batter and shallow fry in hot oil, turning until the batter is cooked

4 Serve with chilli sauce.

This can be made without using the egg (3).

PREPARATION TIME: 10–15 minutes/COOKING TIME: 3–4 minutes for each batch of tempura

VARIATION:
● *Add any firm vegetable to taste, or try shelled prawns with their tail on, squid or pieces of white fish.*

TOMATO CURRY WITH BOILED EGGS (5)
CORE INGREDIENT
4 eggs

FRUIT/VEGETABLES
1 large onion, finely chopped
3–4 cloves garlic, minced
1 T ginger, minced
3 vine-ripened tomatoes, chopped
1 T lemon juice

HERBS AND SPICES
1 red chilli
1 tsp ground coriander
1 tsp ground cumin
1/2 tsp turmeric
1/2 tsp cayenne pepper

1/2 tsp salt or to taste
1 tsp garam masala
fresh coriander

1 Hard boil the eggs, cool them under cold water, shell, cut in half and set aside
2 Heat the oil and stir-fry the onions for 4 to 5 minutes until they turn golden brown
3 Add the garlic, ginger and spices and continue to stir-fry for 1 to 2 minutes then add the tomatoes and salt and continue to fry for another couple of minutes
4 Add the water and simmer until the tomatoes form a thick sauce, stir in the lemon juice and garam masala
5 Add the eggs, garnish with fresh coriander and serve with steamed rice.

PREPARATION TIME: 5 minutes/COOKING TIME: 15–20 minutes

VEGETABLE SUGGESTIONS
● Grilled fennel
● Steamed zucchini tossed in pesto
● Asparagus drizzled with olive oil and chopped chives
● Asparagus served with a poached egg
● Roast peppers

7.4 SENSUOUS SEAFOOD

Seafood, from seaweed to shark, is an important part of the Eastern diet. It is an excellent source of protein, iodine, calcium and other minerals. Coldwater fish such as sardines, mackerel and tuna also contain concentrations of good fats known as omega-3 oils. Fish are rich in vitamin D which is essential for healthy bones and is also thought to help prevent breast cancer.

Fish rather than meat has been a staple food of Japan and Thailand where breast and prostate cancer rates have always been low. Fish is perfect grilled, poached, steamed or fried and served on its own or with a light sauce. There is an infinite variety of fish around at the moment so be adventurous but ensure you buy seafood from the open ocean or freshwater fish and shellfish from rivers that do not have sewage discharges because these can contain harmful chemicals. Tuna, marlin and swordfish are all available at many fish counters. They only need lightly searing and are tough and rubbery if overcooked.

Remember, the Japanese eat all of these fish raw.

BECAUSE FISH COOKS SO QUICKLY IT IS THE ULTIMATE FAST FOOD!

SEAFOOD

BARBECUED SQUID (9)
CORE INGREDIENT
10–12 baby squid

FRUIT/VEGETABLES
2 T lemon or lime juice

FROM THE CUPBOARD
100 gm rice vermicelli
1 T brown sugar
2 tsp fish sauce
2 T olive oil
3 T soya sauce

HERBS AND SPICES
2–3 fresh red chillies, chopped
1 tsp sea salt
1 tsp black pepper
2 T fresh coriander leaves, chopped

1 Combine the chillies, salt and pepper on a plate
2 Wash the squid and dry it well on a paper towel
3 Cut each squid in half and brush them with olive oil and press into the chilli mix to coat both sides

4 Combine the soya sauce, lemon juice, sugar and fish sauce
5 Pour boiling water on to the vermicelli and allow it to stand for 2 to 3 minutes then drain
6 Cook the squid very briefly on each side on a barbecue or griddle pan
7 Pour the soya sauce mixture over the noodles and toss and serve into individual bowls
8 Top with the squid and garnish with fresh coriander leaves.

PREPARATION TIME: 6–8 minutes/COOKING TIME: 2–3 minutes

FISH CAKES (9)
CORE INGREDIENT
125 gm crab meat
250 gm cod or other firm white fish
1 medium egg

FRUIT/VEGETABLES
1 T fresh ginger
2–3 cloves garlic
2 potatoes

FROM THE CUPBOARD
1 T soya milk

HERBS AND SPICES
1 stalk lemon grass
1 red chilli

2 T chopped coriander
salt and pepper to taste

1 Steam or boil the potatoes, drain and mash with a little soya milk
2 Process all the other ingredients in a blender or food processor in short sharp bursts to coarsely flake the fish and season to taste
3 Mix the potato and fish together and mould into burger shapes
4 Shallow fry them until they are cooked through, approximately 5 minutes each side.

PREPARATION TIME: 7–8 minutes/COOKING TIME: 25–30 mins

PRAWNS SAUTÉED WITH FENNEL AND SPINACH (6)
CORE INGREDIENT
450 gm green king or tiger prawns, peeled

FRUIT/VEGETABLES
2 cloves garlic, minced
2 bulbs fennel, sliced
2–3 cups of spinach
1 red pepper, sliced
2 T lemon juice

FROM THE CUPBOARD
2 T olive oil

1/3 cup of Pernod (optional)
2 T dry white wine or mirin

HERBS AND SPICES
salt and pepper to taste
2 T chives, chopped

1 Sauté the garlic, red pepper
and fennel in the olive oil for
about 2 to 3 minutes
2 Add the prawns and wine and
sauté for another 2 to 3 minutes
until the prawns turn pink
3 Add the spinach, Pernod,
lemon juice, chives and
salt/pepper to the pan and sauté
for 1 to 2 minutes until the
spinach is just wilted.

Serve with steamed rice.

PREPARATION TIME:
2–3 minutes/COOKING TIME:
5–6 minutes

SCALLOPS WITH GARLIC AND CORIANDER (9)
CORE INGREDIENT
500 gm small fresh scallops

FRUIT/VEGETABLES
2–3 cloves garlic, chopped
2 T lemon juice

FROM THE CUPBOARD
2 T olive oil

HERBS AND SPICES
salt and pepper
2 T freshly chopped coriander

1 Heat the oil over a low to
medium heat then sauté the
garlic for one minute
2 Add the scallops and lemon
juice, season with salt and
pepper and stir-fry turning
occasionally for about 3 minutes
or until scallops are just cooked
3 Serve with steamed rice and a
green salad.

PREPARATION TIME:
1–2 minutes/COOKING TIME:
5 minutes

STIR-FRIED SQUID (9)
CORE INGREDIENT
500 gm baby squid

FRUIT/VEGETABLES
3–4 cloves garlic, minced
1 onion, chopped
1 T lemon juice

FROM THE CUPBOARD
3 T olive oil

HERBS AND SPICES
1 red chilli, chopped
2 T coriander, chopped
salt and pepper to taste

1 Rinse the squid, pat dry on a paper towel and cut into rings
2 Heat the oil and sauté the onion for 3 to 4 minutes then add the garlic and chilli and continue to sauté for about a minute
3 Add the squid and sauté on a high heat for 2 to 3 minutes until it has all turned opaque
4 Sprinkle with lemon juice and chopped coriander
5 Serve with a green salad and steamed rice.

PREPARATION TIME:
2–3 minutes/COOKING TIME:
5–7 minutes

STIR-FRIED PRAWNS WITH RED PEPPER (6)

Tom Simpson, Jane's youngest son, contributed his simple but delicious stir-fry, which he cooks when home from university.

CORE INGREDIENT
250 gm green prawns, peeled but with the tails left on

FRUIT/VEGETABLES
1 T garlic, minced
2 medium red peppers, sliced
16 small asparagus spears, cut into 3 cm pieces
2 large field mushrooms, sliced
1 T lemon or lime juice

FROM THE CUPBOARD
2 T olive oil

HERBS AND SPICES
fresh coriander
salt and pepper to taste

1 Heat the oil, add the garlic, red pepper, asparagus and mushrooms and stir-fry for 2 to 3 minutes
2 Add the prawns and stir-fry until they turn pink (2 to 3 mins)
3 Season to taste and serve garnished with fresh coriander.

PREPARATION TIME:
2–3 minutes, depending on whether you have to peel the prawns/COOKING TIME:
5–6 minutes

STIR-FRIED PRAWNS WITH SNAP PEAS, SNOWPEAS AND ASPARAGUS (6)

CORE INGREDIENT
300 gm green prawns, peeled

FRUIT/VEGETABLES
3–4 cloves garlic, minced
1 T ginger, minced
16 small asparagus spears, cut into 5cm-length pieces
100 gm snap peas
100 gm snowpeas
1 T lemon or lime juice

FROM THE CUPBOARD
2 T olive oil
1 T sesame seeds or pine nuts
1 T mirin

HERBS AND SPICES
2 T fresh coriander, chopped
salt and pepper to taste

1 Toast the sesame seeds or
pine nuts in a small frying pan
for 1 to 2 minutes
2 Heat the oil, add the garlic,
ginger, snap peas and asparagus
and stir-fry for 2 to 3 minutes
3 Add the prawns and cook
until they just turn pink
4 Add the snowpeas, lemon
juice and mirin and continue to
cook for one minute
5 Season to taste and sprinkle
with sesame seeds or pine nuts
and coriander.

PREPARATION TIME:
1–2 minutes/COOKING TIME:
10 minutes

THAI-STYLE MUSSELS
WITH COCONUT MILK (9)
CORE INGREDIENT
1 kg mussels, live in the shell

FRUIT/VEGETABLES
1 small onion
3–4 cloves garlic
1 T fresh ginger
4–6 spring onions, chopped

1 T lemon or lime juice

FROM THE CUPBOARD
3 T olive oil
1–1¹/₂ cups coconut milk
¹/₄ cup white wine or
 ¹/₄ cup chicken stock
1 T fish sauce

HERBS AND SPICES
2 green chillies
1 stalk lemon grass
4–5 fresh lime leaves
salt and pepper
2–3 T coriander, chopped

1 Clean the mussels by
removing the 'beard' and
washing in cold water. Discard
those that do not close
2 Process the onion, garlic,
ginger, chillies, lemon grass,
lime leaves and two tablespoons
of olive oil in a food processor
until it forms a smooth paste
3 Heat the remaining olive oil,
add the paste and stir-fry for 2
to 3 minutes
4 Slowly add the coconut milk
stirring to mix with the paste,
then mix in the stock and the
fish sauce, and bring to a low
simmer
5 Add the mussels, cover the
pan and cook for about 5 to 7
minutes until the mussels have
opened and are cooked (discard
any that haven't opened)

6 Add the spring onions and lemon juice and continue cooking for another minute
7 Serve in soup bowls sprinkled with chopped coriander.

PREPARATION TIME: 5-6 minutes/COOKING TIME: 10-12 mins

FISH

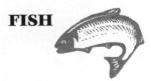

SPICY GRILLED TUNA (9)
CORE INGREDIENT
4 tuna steaks

FRUIT/VEGETABLES
1 T olive oil
2 T lemon juice
2 cloves garlic, chopped
1 T ginger, minced

HERBS AND SPICES
1/2 tsp cumin
2 T fresh coriander
salt and pepper

1 Mix together the olive oil, lemon juice, garlic, ginger and cumin and pour over the tuna and leave to marinate for at least one hour
2 Remove the steaks from the marinade and pat dry, reserving the marinade

3 Grill the tuna steaks on a high heat either on a griddle pan, under the grill or on the barbecue for 3 to 4 minutes each side depending on the thickness of the steaks. They should still be underdone (or even raw) in the middle
4 Heat the marinade in a pan and pour over the fish and sprinkle with fresh coriander.

Serve with a fresh green or nicoise salad.

PREPARATION TIME: 1-2 minutes plus marinating time
COOKING TIME: 6-8 minutes

SWORDFISH BROCHETTES (9)
CORE INGREDIENT
500 kg swordfish, cut into cubes

FRUIT/VEGETABLES
2-3 cloves garlic, chopped
1 T ginger, minced
2 T lemon juice
1 green pepper, coarsely chopped
1 red pepper, coarsely chopped
8 shallots, peeled, halved if large
2 zucchini, cut into chunks
8 cherry tomatoes

FROM THE CUPBOARD
2 T olive oil

HERBS AND SPICES
1 T dried oregano or Italian
herbs or fresh coriander

1 Beat together the olive oil,
lemon juice, garlic, ginger and
herbs and marinate the fish for
at least an hour
2 Thread the vegetables and fish
on to skewers, brush with the
marinade and grill for 5 to 7
minutes each side until just
cooked. Baste with the marinade
whilst cooking to ensure the fish
stays moist.

PREPARATION TIME:
15 minutes, plus 1 hour
marinating/ COOKING TIME:
10–15 minutes

FISH STEW (9)

This is a cross between a soup
and a stew. Serve it with fresh
crusty bread.

CORE INGREDIENT
300 gm firm white fish (cod,
    haddock, monkfish), cut
    into cubes
200 gm mixed seafood (green
    prawns, scallops, mussels,
    squid) in whatever proportions
    you prefer

FRUIT/VEGETABLES
1 onion, chopped
3–4 cloves garlic, chopped

3 medium potatoes, chopped
    into fairly large cubes
3 medium vine-ripened
    tomatoes, chopped
2 cup of fresh or frozen peas
1 cup of small mushrooms
1 T lemon juice

FROM THE CUPBOARD
3 T olive oil
1¼ L fish or vegetable stock
½ cup of white wine (optional)

HERBS AND SPICES
1 red chilli, chopped
½ tsp cumin
1 tsp paprika
2 lime leaves
2 T chopped coriander or
    Italian parsley
1 T chopped chives

1 Wash and clean the mussels,
cut the squid into rings and peel
and de-vein the prawns (the
prawns can be put in whole
which makes the dish look very
interesting)
2 Heat the oil and stir-fry the
onion for 2 to 3 minutes, add
the garlic and chilli and
continue to sauté for another
minute
3 Add the potatoes, cumin,
paprika, lime leaves and a little
salt and pepper and stir-fry for 2
to 3 minutes
4 Add the tomatoes and stock,

bring to the boil, reduce the heat and simmer for about 20 to 30 minutes until the potatoes are soft

5 Add the fish and mushrooms and continue to simmer for about 5 minutes until the fish has changed colour and it is cooked through
6 Add the seafood and peas and simmer for 3 to 4 minutes until the prawns have turned pink and the mussels have opened
7 Stir through the lemon juice and serve garnished with coriander or parsley and chopped chives.

PREPARATION TIME: 10 minutes/COOKING TIME: 30–40 mins

BAKED OCEAN PERCH WITH TOMATOES AND SPINACH (9)
CORE INGREDIENT
4 fillets ocean perch

FRUIT/VEGETABLES
2–3 cloves garlic, chopped
4–5 vine-ripened tomatoes (about 450 gm), sliced
2 cups of spinach
1/2 fennel bulb, sliced

FROM THE CUPBOARD
2 T olive oil
1 T red wine vinegar

HERBS AND SPICES
1/3 cup fresh basil leaves
salt and pepper to taste

1 Bake the fish fillets in the oven for about 15 minutes, until the fish is just cooked
2 Heat the olive oil and sauté the garlic and fennel for 1 to 2 mins
3 Add the tomato, spinach, shredded basil and red wine vinegar and continue to stir-fry until the spinach is just wilted
4 Serve the vegetables on individual plates with the fish on top.

This dish is delicious served with steamed minted baby new potatoes.

PREPARATION TIME: 3–4 minutes/COOKING TIME: 15 minutes

VARIATION:
● *Use any fish and steam, grill or poach to cook*

BARBECUED WHOLE FISH (9)
CORE INGREDIENT
1 whole fish (about 1 kg)

FRUIT/VEGETABLES
6–8 cloves garlic, minced
1 T ginger, minced

2–3 spring onions, chopped
1 T lime juice

FROM THE CUPBOARD
2 T olive oil

HERBS AND SPICES
2 T fresh coriander
2–3 lime leaves, shredded
1 stalk lemon grass, finely
  chopped
salt and pepper to taste

1 Wash and pat dry the fish and put it on a piece of foil large enough to cover the fish
2 Fill the cavity of the fish with spring onions, garlic, ginger, lime leaves, lemon grass and coriander and season with salt and pepper
3 Pour the olive oil and lime juice over the fish
4 Fold over the foil and ensure all the corners are properly sealed so that the juices cannot leak out
5 Place on the barbecue or in the oven and cook for 20 to 30 minutes. If barbecuing, turn the fish over after 10 minutes.

PREPARATION TIME:
3–4 minutes/COOKING TIME:
20–30 minutes

COD WITH OLIVE OIL AND PINE NUTS (9)
CORE INGREDIENT
4 fillets of cod

FRUIT/VEGETABLES
2 cloves garlic, chopped
2 T lemon juice

FROM THE CUPBOARD
3 T olive oil
2 T pine nuts

HERBS AND SPICES
chopped parsley

1 Toast the pine nuts in a pan or in the oven for 3 to 4 minutes until they change colour
2 Heat the olive oil and stir-fry the garlic for one minute
3 Add the lemon juice and the fish and cook for about 4 to 5 minutes turning once
4 Serve garnished with chopped parsley and sprinkled with the pine nuts
5 Serve with a green salad or steamed Asian vegetables.

PREPARATION TIME:
1–2 minutes/COOKING TIME:
7–8 minutes

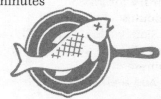

COCONUT AND LIME FISH (9)

CORE INGREDIENT
600 gm firm white fish,
  cut into cubes

FRUIT/VEGETABLES
1 onion, sliced
2–3 cloves garlic, chopped
1 T fresh ginger, sliced
3 T lime or lemon juice

FROM THE CUPBOARD
2 T olive oil
1¹/₂ cups coconut milk
1 tsp fish sauce

HERBS AND SPICES
2 green chillies, chopped
6–8 lime leaves
2 tsp ground cumin
2 tsp ground coriander
1 cinnamon stick
1 star anise
¹/₂ cup of fresh coriander leaves,
  chopped

1 Heat the oil and stir-fry the
onion for 2 to 3 minutes; then
add the ginger, chillies, lime
leaves and all the spices, except
the fresh coriander leaves, and
stir-fry for another 2 to 3
minutes
2 Slowly add the coconut milk
and allow to simmer for about 5
minutes
3 Add the fish and continue to
cook for about 5 minutes or
until the fish is cooked through
4 Add the lime juice and top
with coriander leaves
5 Serve with steamed rice and
bok choy or asparagus in soya
sauce.

PREPARATION TIME:
5–6 minutes/COOKING TIME:
15 minutes

FISH IN COCONUT MILK (9)

CORE INGREDIENT
4 fillets of cod (about 700 gm)

FRUIT/VEGETABLES
1 onion, chopped
4–6 cloves garlic, minced
1 T fresh ginger, minced
1 T lemon juice

FROM THE CUPBOARD
2 T olive oil
400 ml coconut milk
1 tsp fish sauce

HERBS AND SPICES
2 T fresh coriander, chopped
4 lime leaves
1 stick lemon grass, chopped
1 red chilli, sliced
¹/₂ tsp turmeric
salt and pepper to taste

1 Heat the oil and sauté the
onion for 2 to 3 minutes, then

add the garlic, ginger, chilli, lime leaves, lemon grass and turmeric and stir-fry for another 2 to 3 minutes
2 Add the coconut milk and fish and simmer for about 7 to 8 minutes
3 Finally add the fish sauce, lemon juice and salt and pepper to taste
4 Serve with steamed rice, garnished with fresh coriander.

PREPARATION TIME:
2–3 minutes/COOKING TIME:
15 minutes

FLAKED FISH SERVED IN LETTUCE LEAVES (9)
CORE INGREDIENT
750 gm firm white fish fillets
1 egg

FRUIT/VEGETABLES
2–4 cloves garlic, chopped
4 coriander roots (optional)
1 small egg
1 T lemon or lime juice
1 iceberg lettuce

FROM THE CUPBOARD
1 T light soya sauce
30 ml coconut milk
1 T plain flour
3–4 T olive oil
1 tsp fish sauce

HERBS AND SPICES
2 T chilli sauce
1 fresh red chilli
1 cup coriander leaves
salt and pepper

1 Grill the fish until it is just cooked, set aside and when cool mash it with a fork
2 Beat the egg and flour together
3 Add all the remaining ingredients, except the olive oil and lettuce leaves, to the fish and stir in the beaten egg and flour
4 Heat the olive oil in a frying pan and lightly fry the fish mixture until the egg is cooked
5 Serve in iceberg lettuce leaves with extra dishes of chilli sauce and soya sauce on the side.

This is a simplified version of Thai fish cakes. The mixture does not stick together which is why it is served in the lettuce leaves.

PREPARATION TIME:
8–10 minutes/COOKING TIME:
8–10 mins

CHILLING THE 'BURGER' MIXTURE IN THE FRIDGE CAN HELP IT STICK TOGETHER.

SAUTÉED COD WITH TOMATOES, OLIVES AND CAPERS (9)

CORE INGREDIENT
350 gm fresh cod, cut into
  8 pieces

FRUIT/VEGETABLES
2–3 cloves garlic, minced
2 large tomatoes, chopped
8 large olives, stoned and
  chopped

FROM THE CUPBOARD
2 T olive oil
1 T capers
1/4 cup of water

HERBAS AND SPICES
1 red chilli, chopped

1 Heat the olive oil, add garlic, chilli and fish and sauté gently for about 2 to 3 minutes, turn the fish over for another 2 minutes
2 Add the tomatoes, water, capers and chopped olives, mix well and continue to cook for about another 2 to 3 minutes
3 Serve with vegetable mashed potatoes (page 160–1) – delicious!

PREPARATION TIME:
3–4 minutes/COOKING TIME:
6–8 minutes

SHALLOW-FRIED COD WITH CORIANDER (9)

CORE INGREDIENT
600 gm cod fillets

FRUIT/VEGETABLES
1 small onion, finely chopped
3–4 cloves garlic, chopped
  juice of half of a lemon

FROM THE CUPBOARD
2 T olive oil

HERBS AND SPICES
1/4 tsp salt
1/4 tsp pepper
3 T fresh coriander
1 T fresh thyme

1 Stir-fry the onion in olive oil in a frying pan, over medium heat, until the onion starts to soften, add the garlic, and continue frying for another minute
2 Add the cod fillets and shallow fry on medium heat for about 5 minutes, turning once
3 Add the lemon juice, thyme, coriander, salt and pepper, cover and cook for about 2 more minutes. Serve immediately.

PREPARATION TIME:
2–3 minutes/COOKING TIME:
10 minutes

FISH PIE (9)

CORE INGREDIENT
350 gm cod, cut into 3 cm
  squares
100 gm scallops
2 baby squid (about 125 gm),
  cut into rings
8–12 green prawns, peeled

FRUIT/VEGETABLES
2–3 cloves garlic, minced
1 T ginger, minced
1 medium onion, finely chopped
1/2 fennel bulb, sliced
2 vine-ripened tomatoes,
  chopped
1 cup of peas
2 cups of baby spinach
4 spring onions, chopped
1 T lemon or lime juice
4 potatoes, peeled

FROM THE CUPBOARD
2–3 T olive oil
1 heaped T small capers
1 tsp fish sauce
2 T water

HERBS AND SPICES
1 stalk lemon grass, chopped
2–3 lime leaves
1 red chilli, chopped
salt and pepper to taste

1 Boil or steam the potatoes
until they are cooked, then
drain and mash with a little
olive oil, or soya 'butter' and
soya 'milk'
2 Heat the oil and fry the onion
for 1 to 2 minutes then add the
garlic, ginger, fennel, chilli,
lemon grass and lime leaves and
continue to stir-fry for another
minute
3 Add the pieces of cod and fry
for 3 to 4 minutes until cooked
through, then add the chopped
tomatoes and a little salt and
about 1 tablespoon of water,
cover and simmer for 2–3
minutes
4 Add the scallops, squid,
prawns, peas and spinach and
another tablespoon of water and
stir-fry for 1 to 2 minutes until
the prawns have just turned
pink and the spinach is starting
to wilt
5 Add the lemon juice, capers
and fish sauce and mix gently.
Remove from the heat
6 Put the fish mixture into a
baking dish, cover with the
potato and put into an oven
preheated to 180°C for about
15 mins.

PREPARATION TIME:
6–7 minutes/COOKING TIME:
40 minutes

BAKED FISH WITH HERBS (9)

This recipe was given to us by Gill's friend Diana Lampe

CORE INGREDIENT
4 fillets of firm white fish

FRUIT/VEGETABLES
2 cloves garlic, chopped
1 T ginger, chopped
1 T lime juice

FROM THE CUPBOARD
1 T olive oil
1 cup breadcrumbs

HERBS AND SPICES
1 red chilli, chopped (optional)
1 cup mixed fresh herbs, e.g.
  Italian parsley, chives, basil,
  coriander, chopped
salt and pepper to taste

1 Mix breadcrumbs, herbs, chilli, garlic, and olive oil together and divide on top of fish and chill for about 30 minutes
2 Put the fish on a baking tray and place in an oven preheated to 200°C, bake for 15 to 20 minutes until fish is cooked through.

PREPARATION TIME:
2–3 minutes/COOKING TIME:
15–20 mins

MAKE YOUR OWN BREADCRUMBS BY PROCESSING SLICES OF OLD BREAD WITH CRUST REMOVED IN A FOOD PROCESSOR.

BAKED FISH WITH OLIVES, TOMATOES AND POTATOES (9)

CORE INGREDIENT
4 fillets white fish

FRUIT/VEGETABLES
1 onion, sliced
2 large potatoes
3–4 large vine-ripened tomatoes, sliced

FROM THE CUPBOARD
2 T olive oil
1/2 cup black olives, stoned and halved

HERBS AND SPICES
salt and pepper to taste
2 T chopped parsley

1 Preheat the oven to 190°C
2 Boil or steam the potato until it is cooked and then cut into thick slices
3 Cover the base of a large baking tray with a very thin layer of olive oil and put in the fish fillets
4 Add all of the other ingredients with a little more

olive oil and bake in the oven
for about 30 to 35 minutes
5 Serve garnished with chopped
parsley.

PREPARATION TIME:
5 minutes/COOKING TIME:
30–60 minutes

SOLE WITH PESTO AND CAPER SAUCE (9)
CORE INGREDIENT
350 gm fresh fillets of sole
  or plaice

FRUIT/VEGETABLES
3–4 garlic cloves
2 T lemon juice

FROM THE CUPBOARD
3–4 T olive oil
1 heaped T small capers

HERBS AND SPICES
1 cup of fresh basil or coriander
salt and pepper to taste

1 Steam, poach or grill the sole
fillets until they are cooked
2 Purée the garlic, olive oil,
capers, lemon juice and basil
leaves in a food processor and
season to taste
3 Serve the pesto with the fish
or mix it through some cooked
pasta or rice.

PREPARATION TIME:
3–4 minutes/COOKING TIME:
10 minutes

VARIATION:
● *Serve with garlic purée – boil 2
heads of peeled garlic cloves in a
little water or wine until very soft,
purée with olive oil or white wine
and salt and pepper to taste.*

7.5 POULTRY WITH PANACHE

CHICKEN
Chicken (or turkey if you
prefer), providing it is organic
and free range, is one of the best
sources of animal protein.
Chicken in small quantities is
another staple of the Asian diet
and other countries where
breast cancer is low.

CHICKEN AND SPICY TOMATO CASSEROLE (9)
CORE INGREDIENT
4–6 chicken thighs

FRUIT/VEGETABLES
1 small onion, finely chopped
3–4 cloves garlic, sliced
3–4 ripe vine-ripened tomatoes,
  chopped

FROM THE CUPBOARD
2 T olive oil
1/3 cup of dry white or red wine

HERBS AND SPICES
salt and pepper to taste
1 red chilli, chopped (optional)
2-3 T Italian parsley, chopped

1 Wash the chicken and pat dry
on a kitchen towel
2 Heat the oil, add the onion
and chilli and sauté for 2 to 3
minutes
3 Add the garlic and chicken
and brown the thighs on both
sides for 3 to 4 minutes. Season
with salt and pepper
4 Add the wine and simmer for
another 2 to 3 minutes
5 Add the tomatoes, cover and
simmer slowly for about 30
minutes or until the chicken is
tender, stirring occasionally
6 If the casserole becomes too
dry just add a little water.

PREPARATION TIME:
3-4 minutes/COOKING TIME
35-40 mins

CHICKEN SATAY (9)
CORE INGREDIENT
1 kg chicken thighs, cut
  into thin slices

FRUIT/VEGETABLES
2-3 cloves garlic, minced
1 onion, coarsely chopped
1 cucumber, cut into cubes

FROM THE CUPBOARD
2 T olive oil
1/4 cup soya sauce
1/4 cup mirin

HERBS AND SPICES
chilli dipping sauce or
  peanut sauce

1 Whisk together the garlic,
olive oil, soya sauce and mirin
2 Pour the marinade over the
chicken pieces and marinate for
at least two hours, or ideally
overnight
3 Thread the chicken on to
bamboo skewers
4 Grill on the barbecue or under
a grill for 2 to 3 minutes each
side ensuring they do not burn
(do not overcook)
5 Serve with pieces of onion
and cucumber and with chilli
dipping sauce or soya sauce.

SOAK BAMBOO SKEWERS
IN WATER FOR AT LEAST
TWO HOURS TO PREVENT
THEM BURNING

PREPARATION TIME: 30 minutes, plus marinating time
COOKING TIME: 5–6 minutes

CHICKEN WITH MIXED VEGETABLES (6)
CORE INGREDIENT
2–3 chicken breasts

FRUIT/VEGETABLES
3–4 cloves garlic, minced
1 T fresh ginger, minced
8 stalks asparagus
1 carrot
60 gm baby corn
60 gm oyster mushrooms
60 gm snowpeas
60 gm bean sprouts
3 spring onions

FROM THE CUPBOARD
2 T olive or peanut oil
1 T dry sherry or mirin
1 tsp fish sauce
1 tsp sesame oil
1/4 cup of water

HERBS AND SPICES
2 red chillies, chopped
2 T fresh coriander

1 Cut the chicken breasts into thin strips, then put them in a bowl with the ginger and sherry or mirin and leave to marinate for at least an hour
2 Cut the asparagus and spring onions into 3 cm long pieces, julienne the carrot, and halve the mushrooms if they are large
3 Heat the oil, add the chicken, garlic and chillies and sauté for 1 to 2 minutes before adding the corn, asparagus, carrot and mushrooms and sautéing for another minute
4 Add the water, bring to the boil, cover and simmer for 2 to 3 mins
5 Add the fish sauce, sesame oil, snowpeas and bean sprouts and stir-fry for 1 to 2 minutes until the vegetables are just cooked
6 Serve garnished with fresh coriander.

PREPARATION TIME: 6–7 minutes, plus marinating time
COOKING TIME: 8–10 minutes

CHICKEN WITH OLIVES AND TOMATO (9)
CORE INGREDIENT
2–3 chicken breasts, sliced

FRUIT/VEGETABLES
1 small onion, finely chopped
3–4 cloves garlic, minced
6–10 kalamata olives, pitted and chopped
3–4 fresh tomatoes, chopped

FROM THE CUPBOARD
3 T olive oil
2 T capers
1/4 cup red wine

HERBS AND SPICES
1/2 tsp salt
1 red chilli, chopped
2 T fresh coriander

1 Stir-fry the onion in the olive oil in a saucepan or wok, over a medium heat, for 2 to 3 minutes
2 Add the chicken, garlic, chilli and olives and continue stir-frying for another 2 to 3 minutes
3 Add the capers, wine, tomatoes and salt and simmer on a low heat for about 5 minutes until the chicken is cooked through
4 Serve garnished with coriander.

PREPARATION TIME:
3–4 minutes/COOKING TIME:
10 minutes

CHICKEN WITH RED CABBAGE (6)
CORE INGREDIENT
4–5 chicken thighs, quartered

FRUIT/VEGETABLES
1 red onion, sliced
1 red cabbage, finely sliced
1 apple, peeled, cored and sliced
3–4 cloves garlic, chopped

FROM THE CUPBOARD
5 T olive oil
1/2 cup of red wine or water

HERBS AND SPICES
salt and pepper

1 Heat 4 tablespoons of oil and sauté the onion for 2 to 3 minutes, before adding the garlic and sautéing for another minute
2 Add the red cabbage, stirring thoroughly to coat the cabbage with the oil
3 Add the wine, season to taste, cover and simmer on a low heat for about 45 minutes adding the sliced apple after about 30 minutes of cooking
4 In a separate pan brown the chicken thighs on both sides in one tablespoon of oil
5 Add them to the cabbage and continue to simmer for another 10–15 minutes or until the chicken is cooked through and tender.

Serve with couscous or polenta.

PREPARATION TIME:
3–5 minutes/COOKING TIME:
60 minutes

CHICKEN WITH RICE (9)
CORE INGREDIENT
4 chicken breasts

FRUIT/VEGETABLES
1 small onion, chopped
2–3 T garlic, minced

2–3 T ginger, minced
4–6 spring onions finely
chopped

FROM THE CUPBOARD
1 T olive oil
1 cup of basmati rice
1¹/₂ litres chicken stock
4 T mirin
2 tsp sugar

HERBS AND SPICES
chilli sauce to serve
2 T chopped coriander

1 Put the garlic and ginger in
separate bowls and add 1
tablespoon of mirin and 1
teaspoon of sugar to each
2 Heat the oil and stir-fry the
onion for 1 to 2 minutes, add
the garlic and rice and continue
frying for another minute
3 Add 2 cups of chicken stock,
season to taste, cover and
simmer for about 12 to 13
minutes until the rice is cooked
4 At the same time poach or
steam the chicken breast until it
is cooked, then slice it and serve
on individual plates
5 Add the remaining stock to a
saucepan, warm through, add
the spring onions and sprinkle
with coriander leaves
6 Serve each person with an
individual plate of chicken, a
bowl of rice, a bowl of soup and

side dishes of garlic, ginger and
chilli sauce.

This meal is typically Asian.
The way to eat it is for each
person to add garlic, ginger and
chilli to taste to each spoonful of
rice or soup.

PREPARATION TIME:
2–3 minutes/COOKING TIME:
15–20 mins

GREEN CURRY CHICKEN (9)
CORE INGREDIENT
6–8 chicken thighs, skinned,
boned and cut into cubes

FRUIT/VEGETABLES
3 shallots
3–4 cloves garlic
2 T ginger or galangal
8–12 oyster mushrooms
100 gm green beans
¹/₂ aubergine, diced
¹/₂ cup of bamboo shoots
¹/₂ cup of baby corn
6–8 stalks asparagus
2–3 spring onions, chopped
2 T lime juice
¹/₂ cup of bean sprouts

FROM THE CUPBOARD
2 T olive oil
2 T water
1 tsp shrimp paste
1 cup of coconut milk

HERBS AND SPICES
3 sticks lemon grass
1 cup of fresh coriander
1/2 tsp cumin
1/4 tsp turmeric
3 green chillies
2–3 lime leaves
6–8 Thai basil leaves

1 Process the shallots, garlic, lemon grass, olive oil, water, shrimp paste, coriander, cumin, turmeric, chillies and lime leaves to a smooth paste in a food processor
2 Stir-fry the paste in a saucepan for 1 to 2 minutes before adding the coconut milk. Bring to a slow simmer and add the chicken, beans and aubergine and simmer for 6 to 7 minutes
3 Add the mushrooms, asparagus, baby corn and bamboo shoots and simmer for another 3–4 minutes until the vegetables are just cooked
4 Stir in the spring onions, bean sprouts and lime juice
5 Serve garnished with Thai basil.

PREPARATION TIME:
10 minutes/COOKING TIME:
15 minutes

SHORT CUT: Packaged green curry paste can be used.

MINCED CHICKEN IN LETTUCE LEAVES (9)
CORE INGREDIENT
3 chicken breasts, minced

FRUIT/VEGETABLES
3–4 cloves garlic, chopped
1 T ginger, minced
1/3 cup of lemon or lime juice
6 spring onions
1 green pepper, finely chopped
2 cups of spinach
8 large lettuce leaves

FROM THE CUPBOARD
2 T olive or peanut oil
2 T soya sauce
1 tsp fish sauce

HERBS AND SPICES
1 red chilli, chopped
1 cup of chopped fresh mint
  and coriander or basil
salt and pepper

1 Heat the oil, add the garlic, ginger, pepper and chilli and fry for 1 to 2 minutes
2 Add the chicken and stir-fry for 3 to 4 minutes until the chicken is cooked through
3 Add the rest of the ingredients, except the lettuce leaves, mix well and cook until the spinach just wilts. Season to taste
4 Serve in the lettuce leaves and eat with fingers after folding the

lettuce around the chicken mixture.

PREPARATION TIME:
5–8 minutes/COOKING TIME:
8–10 minutes

MINCED CHICKEN WITH GREEN BEANS AND RED PEPPER (6)
CORE INGREDIENT
3 chicken breasts or thighs, minced

FRUIT/VEGETABLES
6 cloves garlic, minced
1 red pepper, sliced
500 gm green beans cut
  into 3 cm pieces

FROM THE CUPBOARD
2 T olive oil
1/2 cup of water
1 tsp fish sauce

HERBS AND SPICES
1 red chilli, chopped
1/2 tsp paprika

1 Heat the oil and add all the ingredients except the water to the pan and stir-fry for 1 to 2 minutes
2 Add the water, cover the pan and cook until the beans are tender – about 3 to 4 minutes.

PREPARATION TIME:
3–4 minutes/COOKING TIME:
5–6 minutes

VARIATION:
● *Use minced pork instead of the chicken.*

ROAST PAPRIKA CHICKEN WITH LEMONS (9)
Emma Simpson, Jane's daughter, contributed this simple elegant recipe for a really moist roast chicken.

CORE INGREDIENT
1 1/2 kg whole chicken

FRUIT/VEGETABLES
2 lemons

FROM THE CUPBOARD
1 T olive oil

HERBS AND SPICES
1 T paprika
1 tsp salt

1 Wash the chicken inside and out and pat dry with kitchen paper
2 Mix together the salt, paprika and olive oil and brush over the entire chicken
3 Prick the lemons all over and put them into the chicken cavity
4 Put the chicken in a baking tray breast side down and roast

in a preheated 180°C oven for about 30 minutes. Turn the chicken over and continue to roast for another 30 minutes. Finally, turn the heat up to 200°C for another 20–30 minutes

5 Serve on a meat dish garnished with fresh watercress.

PREPARATION TIME:
2–3 minutes/COOKING TIME:
1½ hours

SPICY CHICKEN AND TOMATO CURRY (9)
CORE INGREDIENT
8 chicken thighs

FRUIT/VEGETABLES
1 large onion, sliced
3 medium tomatoes, chopped
1 T ginger, chopped
1 T garlic, chopped
6 spring onions, chopped
1 T lemon juice

FROM THE CUPBOARD
3 T olive oil
¼ cup water

HERBS AND SPICES
5–6 cloves
1 cinnamon stick
3 star anise
1 tsp salt
2 tsp cayenne pepper
  (or to taste)

½ tsp turmeric
1 tsp cumin
2 tsp coriander
mint or coriander to garnish

1 Heat the oil and fry the onions, star anise, cloves and cinnamon stick for 2 to 3 minutes then add the garlic and ginger and the rest of the spices and fry for another 1 to 2 minutes

2 Add the chicken and stir-fry until well coated with the spices and browned

3 Add the chopped tomatoes and water and simmer until the chicken is tender – about 20 minutes

4 Serve with chopped spring onions, mint leaves and lemon juice.

Any leftovers are excellent reheated and served with salad.

PREPARATION TIME:
5–6 minutes/COOKING TIME:
20–25 minutes

STIR-FRIED CHICKEN IN BLACK PEPPER (9)
CORE INGREDIENT
4–6 chicken thighs, skinned and
  boned and cut into chunks

FRUIT/VEGETABLES
1 green pepper, sliced

1 red pepper, sliced
1 cup green peas
3–4 cloves garlic, chopped
1 T ginger, minced

FROM THE CUPBOARD
2 T olive oil

HERBS AND SPICES
1–2 T coarse black pepper
1 tsp salt
2 T fresh coriander

1 Mix together the garlic, ginger, pepper and salt, add the chicken, stir to coat with the mixture and leave for at least 20 minutes
2 Heat the olive oil, add the chicken and spices and stir-fry for 5 to 6 minutes, then add the green and red pepper and continue to cook for another 2 to 3 minutes
3 Finally add the peas and heat through
4 Serve with steamed rice and garnish with fresh coriander.

PREPARATION TIME: 5 minutes and 20 minutes standing
COOKING TIME: 10–12 minutes

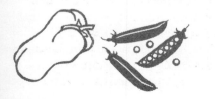

STIR-FRIED CHICKEN WITH MUSHROOMS AND BEAN SPROUTS (6)
This can be served hot with rice or prepared with raw vegetables as a salad.

CORE INGREDIENT
2–3 chicken breasts, sliced

FRUIT/VEGETABLES
125 gm mushrooms, sliced
2 cups bean sprouts
2 cloves garlic, minced
4–5 spring onions, sliced

FROM THE CUPBOARD
1 T olive oil
1 T sesame oil
2 T soya sauce

HERBS AND SPICES
1 red chilli, chopped (optional)
1/2 tsp black pepper
2 T chopped fresh herbs –
    chives, parsley, basil or
    coriander

1 Heat the olive oil and fry the garlic and chilli for one minute
2 Add the chicken and continue to fry for 3 to 4 minutes before adding the mushrooms and soya sauce and frying for another 2 to 3 minutes
3 Add the sesame oil, bean sprouts, spring onions and black pepper and continue to cook for

another minute
4 Serve garnished with chopped herbs of your choice.

PREPARATION TIME:
5 minutes/COOKING TIME:
10 minutes

VARIATION:
● *Cook the chicken, serve the vegetables raw mixed with the herbs and pour over the dressing made from the garlic, chilli, sesame oil, olive oil and soya sauce.*

TANDOORI-STYLE CHICKEN THIGHS (9)
CORE INGREDIENT
1½ kg chicken thighs

FRUIT/VEGETABLES
1 tsp fresh ginger
1 tsp fresh garlic
2 T lemon juice

FROM THE CUPBOARD
3 T olive or peanut oil
3 T unsweetened plain soya 'yoghurt'

HERBS AND SPICES
1½ tsp ground cumin
1½ tsp ground coriander
1 tsp cayenne pepper
1 tsp paprika
1 tsp salt

1 Mix together all the ingredients except the chicken thighs and soya yoghurt in a food processor and process to a smooth paste
2 Mix equal proportions of 'yoghurt' and the paste (enough to fully coat the thighs). Add the chicken thighs, stir well and marinate for at least 24 hours in the fridge (they can be left for up to 2 days)
3 Barbecue, roast or grill the chicken in the oven for about 25 minutes (check that they are thoroughly cooked).
These are delicious cold so it is as well to cook plenty and use the leftovers for picnics or packed lunches.

PREPARATION TIME: 5 minutes plus 24 hours for marinating
COOKING TIME: 25 minutes

SHORT CUT: Use prepared tikka or tandoori paste.

DUCK
Duck is another staple of the Asian diet. In China ducks are used to gobble up snails in the paddy fields, a practice which helps to reduce serious waterborne diseases.

Do not eat duck skin, because any man-made hormone-mimicking chemicals that are around tend to concentrate in the fatty layer just under the skin. Also, for this reason do not use the duck fat to cook roast potatoes.

DUCK IN CHINESE PANCAKES (9)

CORE INGREDIENT
1 Gressingham duck or 3–4 duck breasts

FRUIT/VEGETABLES
8 spring onions, julienned
1 cucumber, julienned
1 cup bean sprouts

FROM THE CUPBOARD
1 packet Chinese pancakes
plum sauce or Hoisin sauce to serve
1 T olive oil

HERBS AND SPICES
1 tsp salt
1 tsp paprika
chilli sauce to serve

1 Mix together the salt, paprika and olive oil
2 Wash and pat dry the duck and put it in the fridge to dry the skin for about 30 minutes, then brush it with the olive oil mixture
3 Place the duck on a rack in a baking tray and roast in an oven preheated to 200°C for about an hour until the duck is well cooked. Make sure there is plenty of space between the rack and the bottom of the baking tray, or drain off the duck fat during cooking
4 Remove the duck from the oven and allow it to stand for about 10 minutes, before carving into small pieces on a serving plate
5 Steam the pancakes for about 3 to 4 minutes until they are warmed through
6 Put the pancakes, the plate of duck, individual plates of bean sprouts, spring onions, cucumber, hoisin sauce and chilli sauce on the table.

PREPARATION TIME:
10 minutes/COOKING TIME:
60 minutes

Each person helps themselves to a pancake, spreads a little of the hoisin sauce down the centre, adds a few pieces of the duck, some spring onion, bean sprouts and cucumber and a little chilli sauce to taste and rolls up the pancake to eat with their fingers.

SHORT CUT: A good short cut is to buy duck breast marinated in Chinese sauce. Cook for about 40 minutes and shred before serving.

SPICED DUCK WITH BOK CHOY (6)
CORE INGREDIENT
2-3 duck breasts, skinned

FRUIT/VEGETABLES
2 cloves garlic, minced
2 T lemon juice
4 baby bok choy, halved

FROM THE CUPBOARD
1 tsp olive oil
1 tsp soya sauce

HERBS AND SPICES
2 tsp ground cumin
1 tsp ground coriander
2 tsp chilli sauce

1 Mix together the garlic, lemon juice, olive oil, soya sauce, cumin, coriander and chilli sauce and put in a baking dish
2 Add the duck; ensure it is well coated with the sauce and leave it to marinate for at least 30 minutes
3 Bake the duck in a preheated 170°C oven for about 40 minutes
4 Steam the bok choy for about 5 to 7 minutes until just tender

5 Slice the duck finely and serve on the steamed bok choy and sprinkle with extra soya sauce.

PREPARATION TIME: 3–4 minutes, plus at least 30 minutes marinating/COOKING TIME: 40 minutes

EGGS

POTATO TORTILLA (8)
CORE INGREDIENT
4 eggs

FRUIT/VEGETABLES
2 large potatoes
1 large onion, sliced
3-4 cloves garlic, finely chopped

FROM THE CUPBOARD
2 T olive oil
1 T water

HERBS AND SPICES
salt and pepper
2 T chopped parsley
1 T chopped chives

1 Parboil or steam the potatoes, then drain them and cut into thin slices
2 Sprinkle a little salt over the potatoes and onions
3 Heat the oil and add the garlic, potato and onions. Cook slowly over a medium heat

stirring occasionally until the potatoes are soft but not brown
4 Lightly beat the eggs with the water, season to taste and gently stir in the parsley and chives
5 Pour the egg mixture over the potatoes
6 Cook, shaking the pan occasionally to stop the mixture sticking. When the underside has browned either turn the tortilla over in the pan or put it under the grill to finish cooking the top.
7 Serve with a salad.

PREPARATION TIME:
6–7 minutes/COOKING TIME:
20 minutes

ONION AND MUSHROOM FRITTATA (8)
CORE INGREDIENT
4 eggs

FRUIT/VEGETABLES
4 small to medium onions, finely sliced
3–4 cloves garlic, chopped
125 gm chestnut mushrooms, sliced

FROM THE CUPBOARD
3–4 T olive oil
1 T water

HERBS AND SPICES
3 T chopped parsley
salt and pepper to taste

1 Heat the oil, add the onions and a little salt, and sauté on a low heat until the onions become deep golden brown and are very soft
2 In a separate saucepan fry the mushrooms for 2 to 3 minutes
3 Beat the eggs with the water
4 Add the mushrooms and the chopped parsley to the onions (if you think there is too much oil in the onions drain it off) and stir together gently
5 Pour the beaten egg over the mushrooms and cook until the underside is done, then finish off the top under the grill.

PREPARATION TIME:
6–7 minutes/COOKING TIME:
20 minutes

FRITTATA SUGGESTIONS (8)
● Sweet potato or pumpkin frittata
● Green bean frittata
● Roast vegetable frittata
● Asparagus frittata

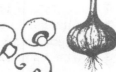
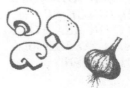

7.6 MEATS – NOW AND THEN

Never buy meat that has been treated with hormones or is from animals which have been used for dairying. Question your butcher thoroughly on these points.

REMEMBER THAT COOKING MEAT SO THAT IT IS BURNED ON THE OUTSIDE AND RAW ON THE INSIDE IS BAD FOR HEALTH. CANCER-FORMING CHEMICALS FORM IN THE BURNT PARTS AND HORMONES AND GROWTH FACTORS REMAIN INTACT IN THE RAW MEAT INSIDE. NEVER FLAMBÉ OR BURN MEATS OR FISH AND NEVER RE-USE COOKING OILS ESPECIALLY IF THEY HAVE BEEN USED TO COOK MEAT OR FISH.

NEVER BUY MINCED MEAT (LAMB, PORK, CHICKEN). ALWAYS CHOOSE A GOOD CUT AND MINCE IT YOURSELF OR ASK YOUR BUTCHER TO MINCE IT FOR YOU.

LAMB

If you want to eat lamb, ensure you always buy young meat.

CURRIED MINCED LAMB WITH CORIANDER (10)
CORE INGREDIENT
450 gm lamb, minced

FRUIT/VEGETABLES
1 large onion, finely chopped
4–6 cloves garlic, finely chopped
1 cup peas
1 T lemon juice

FROM THE CUPBOARD
2 T olive oil
1/2 cup water or stock

HERBS AND SPICES
1/2 tsp salt
1 1/2 tsp ground cumin
1 1/2 tsp ground coriander
1 1/2 tsp cayenne powder
3–4 T chopped fresh coriander
1–2 T chopped fresh mint

1 Stir-fry the onion in olive oil in a saucepan for 2 to 3 minutes until the onion is soft, add the garlic and continue stir-frying for another minute.
2 Add the salt, coriander, cumin and cayenne pepper and stir-fry for another 1 to 2 minutes.
3 Add the lamb and stir-fry until it is well browned
4 Add the water, bring to the

boil then cover the pan and simmer stirring occasionally for about 20 minutes, until the lamb is tender

5 After about 15 minutes, add the peas. If the dish is becoming too dry add a little more water

6 Finely chop the coriander and mint together and add to the lamb with the lemon juice just before serving.

PREPARATION TIME: 6–7 minutes/COOKING TIME: 25 minutes

GRILLED MINCED LAMB WITH SPINACH (10)

CORE INGREDIENT
450 gm lamb, minced

FRUIT/VEGETABLES
1 medium onion, sliced
3–4 cloves garlic, minced
1 T ginger, minced
4–6 spring onions, chopped
1 cup of peas
2 cups of spinach
1 small red onion, cut into rings
1 T lemon juice
1 lemon, cut into wedges

FROM THE CUPBOARD
2 T olive oil
1/2 cup of water or stock
2 T soya yoghurt

HERBS AND SPICES
1/2 tsp salt
2–3 green chillies
1 tsp ground coriander
11/2 tsp garam masala
1 tsp cayenne pepper
1/2 bunch fresh coriander, finely chopped

1 Mix the minced lamb with the garlic, ginger, soya 'yoghurt', salt, garam masala, cayenne pepper and ground coriander and one tablespoon olive oil and leave to marinate

2 Heat the remainder of the oil and fry the onion until it is golden brown, about 4 to 5 minutes

3 Add the lamb and spices and stir-fry for 10 to 15 minutes until the lamb is well cooked

4 Add the spring onions, peas and spinach and cook until the spinach is just wilted and the peas are warmed through

5 Add the fresh coriander and green chillies and stir into the meat with the lemon juice

6 Transfer to a baking dish and place under the grill or in the oven for 10 to 15 minutes. If grilling stir occasionally to prevent the lamb burning

7 Serve garnished with red onion rings and lemon wedges.

PREPARATION TIME:
5 minutes/COOKING TIME:
30-35 minutes

MINCED LAMB 'BURGERS' WITH TAHINI SAUCE (10)

CORE INGREDIENT
450 gm lamb, minced

FRUIT/VEGETABLES
2 medium onions, chopped
3-4 cloves garlic, chopped
2 T lemon juice

FROM THE CUPBOARD
3 T olive oil
1/2 cup cracked wheat
3 T pine nuts
4 T tahini paste
1/4 cup water

HERBS AND SPICES
1 cup parsley, finely chopped
1 T ground cumin
1 tsp garam masala
1/2 tsp ground nutmeg
salt and pepper to taste

1 Soak the cracked wheat in cold water for 10 to 15 minutes then drain
2 Mix the wheat with the minced lamb, onions, garlic, parsley, salt, spices and pine nuts
3 Make the lamb into smallish burgers, about 5 cm across, and shallow fry in the oil at a medium temperature, until they are cooked through
4 Whisk together the tahini, water and lemon juice
5 Heat the tahini sauce gently and pour over the burger.

PREPARATION TIME:
10 minutes, plus 15 minutes soaking/ COOKING TIME:
10-15 minutes

BARBECUED SPICED LEG OF LAMB (10)

Ask your butcher to butterfly a leg of lamb for you (remove the bone and open it up).

CORE INGREDIENT
1 leg of lamb, butterflied

FRUIT/VEGETABLES
2 medium onions
3 cm ginger
7-8 cloves garlic
1/2 cup of lemon juice

FROM THE CUPBOARD
1/2 cup of olive oil

HERBS AND SPICES
1 1/2 T cayenne pepper
1 T ground coriander
1 T ground cumin
1 T garam masala
1/4 tsp nutmeg
1/4 tsp cinnamon
4 cloves

2 1/2 tsp salt
1 T coarsely ground black
  pepper

1 Process all ingredients except
the lamb in a food processor to
make a smooth paste
2 Make jabs in the lamb with a
sharp knife, put in a large
mixing bowl and cover with the
paste. Cover and refrigerate for
at least 24 hours
3 Barbecue or bake the lamb in
an oven until cooked to your
liking, approximately 45
minutes on the barbeque, or 60
minutes in the oven depending
on the size of the leg.

PREPARATION TIME:
5–6 minutes/COOKING TIME:
45–60 minutes

LAMB AND SPINACH CURRY (10)
CORE INGREDIENT
1 kg leg of lamb, cubed

FRUIT/VEGETABLES
2 large onions, finely chopped
6 cloves garlic, chopped
500 gm fresh spinach
3–4 large vine-ripened
  tomatoes, chopped

FROM THE CUPBOARD
3 T olive oil

HERBS AND SPICES
1 T ground cumin
1/2 T ground coriander
1 tsp cayenne pepper
1 tsp salt
2 cups of fresh coriander

1 Heat the oil and stir-fry the
onions over a medium to low
heat until they become light
brown. Add the garlic and
continue frying for another
minute
2 Add the salt, ground
coriander, cumin and cayenne
pepper and fry for another 2
minutes, then add the lamb and
brown it on all sides
3 Chop the spinach and one cup
of coriander with the stalks in a
food processor and add to the
lamb
4 Finely chop the tomatoes in
the food processor and add to
the lamb and spinach. Simmer,
covered, for about 45 minutes.
Stir occasionally to make sure it
doesn't stick, and add water if it
becomes too dry
5 Serve, sprinkled with extra
fresh coriander leaves.

PREPARATION TIME:
10 minutes/COOKING TIME:
50 minutes

This dish can be returned to the
fridge, when cool, and

re-heated. Like a good wine it actually improves after a few days!

LAMB AND GREEN OLIVE TAPENADE (10)
CORE INGREDIENT
2 lamb loins (1½ to 2 kilos; filleted by your butcher)

FROM THE CUPBOARD
275–300 gm green olive paste/marinade, or tapenade
2 T olive oil

1 Mix the olive paste with the olive oil
2 Place the lamb loins on a baking tray, cover with the olive paste and leave to marinate for at least 30 minutes
3 Barbecue or roast the lamb in the oven for about 25 minutes (you will need to watch) depending on the heat and size of the loins.

Serve with green beans with garlic, mixed green salad and (our favourite) spicy cumin potatoes.

PREPARATION TIME:
2–3 minutes, plus 15 minutes marinating time/COOKING TIME: 25–30 minutes

This is adjusted easily for any number of people. Any left over is delicious served cold for lunch the next day.

LAMB WITH GREEN PEPPER (10)
CORE INGREDIENT
1 kg leg of lamb, cubed

FRUIT/VEGETABLES
1 large onion, coarsely sliced
3 tsp ginger, minced
3 tsp garlic, minced
4–5 fresh tomatoes, chopped
2 green peppers, chopped
1 T lemon juice

FROM THE CUPBOARD
3 T olive oil
½ cup water
½ cup coconut milk

HERBS AND SPICES
2 long green chillies
1 cinnamon stick
5–6 cloves
4 cardamom pods, crushed
3 star anise
7–8 curry leaves or 3 bay leaves
1 tsp chilli powder
3 tsp curry powder
½ tsp turmeric
1 tsp salt
mint or coriander for garnish

1 Heat the oil in a large saucepan and fry the onion with the cinnamon stick, green chillies, cloves, cardamoms, star anise and curry leaves for 3 to 4 minutes

2 Add garlic and ginger and all the other spices, except the mint or coriander, and stir-fry for another 1 to 2 minutes

3 Add the lamb in batches and stir until it is well browned

4 Slowly add the water and the chopped tomatoes. Bring to the boil, lower the temperature, and simmer for 20 to 30 minutes uncovered

5 Add the coconut milk and simmer for another 10 minutes

6 Add the diced green pepper, and simmer for another 10 minutes. Add the lemon juice and chopped mint just before serving.

PREPARATION TIME:
5 minutes/COOKING TIME:
50–60 minutes

USE A MEAT
THERMOMETER FOR
ROASTS UNTIL
YOU HAVE ENOUGH
EXPERIENCE NOT TO
NEED ONE. THEY HELP
TO ENSURE THE MEAT IS
THOROUGHLY, BUT NOT
OVER, COOKED.

PORK

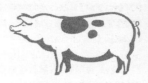

ROAST PORK LOIN
WITH APPLE (10)
CORE INGREDIENT
300 gm pork fillet or 4 pork
  loin chops

FRUIT/VEGETABLES
2 cloves garlic, finely chopped
1 green apple
1 T lemon juice

FROM THE CUPBOARD
2 T olive oil
2 T Calvados (optional)

HERBS AND SPICES
black pepper

1 Marinate the pork in the olive oil, garlic and lemon juice for at least 30 minutes

2 Slice the apple and place in the bottom of a baking dish, put the pork on top, pour over the marinade and Calvados and bake in a preheated 200°C oven for about 10 to 15 minutes. Do not overcook.

PREPARATION TIME:
2–3 minutes/COOKING TIME:
10–15 minutes

STIR-FRIED PORK WITH BOK CHOY (7)
CORE INGREDIENT
300 gm pork fillet, sliced

FRUIT/VEGETABLES
1 onion, coarsely chopped
2 T ginger, minced
3-4 cloves garlic, minced
4 small bok choy, halved
100 gm bean sprouts
4-6 spring onions, chopped
10-12 oyster mushrooms, halved

FROM THE CUPBOARD
2 tsp sesame oil
2 tsp olive oil
2 T Chinese cooking wine
  or mirin
3 T soya sauce

HERBS AND SPICES
1 tsp chilli sauce (optional)

1 Heat the olive oil and sauté the onion for 2 to 3 minutes
2 Add the garlic, ginger, chilli and sliced pork and sauté for 3 to 4 minutes until cooked through
3 Add the mushrooms, spring onions, bok choy, sesame oil, Chinese cooking wine and soya sauce and simmer for 2 to 3 minutes until the vegetables are just tender.
4 Serve with steamed rice.

PREPARATION TIME:
5-6 minutes/COOKING TIME:
10 minutes

RABBIT

ROAST RABBIT WITH TOMATOES AND FENNEL (10)
CORE INGREDIENT
4-8 rabbit portions

FRUIT/VEGETABLES
1 large onion, chopped
4-6 cloves garlic, minced
4-5 tomatoes, chopped
1 large fennel bulb, sliced

FROM THE CUPBOARD
3-4 T olive oil
3-4 T balsamic vinegar
2 T fennel seeds (optional)

HERBS AND SPICES
1 tsp turmeric
1 tsp chopped rosemary
salt and pepper

1 Heat the olive oil in a frying pan or wok and sauté the rabbit portions until brown, then place them in a baking dish and set aside
2 Add the onion to the oil and sauté for 2 to 3 minutes, then add the garlic and fennel and sauté for another 2 minutes
3 Add the tomatoes, turmeric,

rosemary, fennel seed and balsamic vinegar, season to taste and sauté for another minute

4 Pour the sauce over the rabbit and bake in a preheated 180°C oven for about 40 minutes. Halfway through cooking, baste the rabbit adding another tablespoon of balsamic vinegar if necessary

5 Serve with polenta and some green beans.

PREPARATION TIME: 5 minutes/COOKING TIME: 45–50 minutes

RABBIT STEW (10)
CORE INGREDIENT
4–8 rabbit portions

FRUIT/VEGETABLES
1 large onion, sliced
4 cloves garlic, chopped
1 carrot, sliced
1 celery stick, sliced
2 zucchini, sliced
1/2 pumpkin, cubed
1 sweet potato, cubed
2–3 tomatoes, chopped

FROM THE CUPBOARD
4 T olive oil
1/2 cup of white wine
2 T tomato paste
1/2 cup of chicken or vegetable stock
1 can cannellini beans

HERBS AND SPICES
2 tsp rosemary
salt and pepper

1 Marinate the rabbit in olive oil and white wine ideally overnight or for at least 8 hours. Drain and reserve the marinade
2 Heat the oil in a large sauté pan, add the garlic and rabbit and brown
3 Add all the vegetables, tomato paste, stock, marinade and herbs, cover the pan and simmer slowly, turning the rabbit occasionally, for about 45 minutes or until the rabbit is tender
4 Take off the cover and simmer rapidly to reduce some of the liquid
5 Finally, add the cannellini beans, season to taste and continue to simmer for another 15 minutes
6 Serve with polenta or mashed potatoes.

PREPARATION TIME: 15 minutes, plus marinating time/ COOKING TIME: 1 1/4 –1 1/2 hours

VENISON
Venison, kangaroo and ostrich meat is from animals that are kept in free-range conditions, or are not intensively farmed.

They generally have much lower fat and cholesterol levels and are therefore healthier to eat than beef.

SAUTÉED VENISON STEAKS (10)
CORE INGREDIENT
4 good quality venison steaks

FRUIT/VEGETABLES
1 large onion, sliced
3–4 cloves garlic, chopped
100 gm dried shitake
  mushrooms
100 gm flat or chestnut
  mushrooms, sliced

FROM THE CUPBOARD
3 T olive oil
1/2 cup of red wine

HERBS AND SPICES
1 T black pepper
1 T chopped rosemary

1 Marinate the venison steaks in 2 tablespoons olive oil and the red wine for at least one hour, turning occasionally to ensure the meat is well marinated
2 Soak the shitake mushrooms in 1 cup of boiling water for about 30 minutes
3 Transfer the steaks and the marinade into a pan and fry until cooked (10 to 15 minutes).

Alternatively they can be cooked in an oven preheated to 180°C for about 15 to 20 minutes
4 Heat the remaining olive oil in a frying pan and sauté the onions for 2 to 3 minutes then add the garlic, the drained shitake mushrooms with half their liquid, the chestnut mushrooms and plenty of black pepper and simmer until the mushrooms are cooked
5 Serve the steaks, pour the mushroom sauce over them and garnish with chopped rosemary.

PREPARATION TIME: 2–3 minutes, plus marinating time
COOKING TIME: 15–20 minutes

VENISON IN RED WINE (10)
CORE INGREDIENT
1 kg venison, cut into 5 cm
  cubes

FRUIT/VEGETABLES
12–16 shallots
5–6 cloves garlic, minced
12–16 small mushrooms
1–2 parsnips, cubed
2 carrots, sliced

FROM THE CUPBOARD
3–4 T olive oil
2 cups red wine
2 T plain flour
2 cups beef stock

HERBS AND SPICES
pepper
2 bay leaves
2 sprigs thyme
2 T parsley

1 Preheat the oven to 180°C
2 Marinate the venison in 3 to 4
tablespoons of olive oil and 1/2
cup of red wine for at least one
hour. Drain, reserving the
marinade and pat it dry on a
kitchen towel
3 In a casserole dish heat the
oil, brown the onions and set
them aside
4 Add the carrots and parsnips
to the pan and stir-fry for 2 to 3
minutes and set aside with the
onions
5 Add the venison to the pan in
batches and seal the meat,
removing each batch to make
room for the rest of the meat
6 Pour off any fat from the
casserole dish, return the meat
to the pan and add the flour
stirring well for 1 to 2 minutes
7 Add the vegetables, garlic,
marinade, stock and extra red
wine, bay leaves, thyme and
pepper and cook in the oven for
2 hours (check to determine if
the meat is tender – if not
continue cooking for another
30 to 60 minutes)
8 Add the mushrooms and
continue to cook for another

30 minutes
9 If the casserole liquid is a
little thin, heat the casserole on
the top of the stove, mix 2
tablespoons of plain flour with 1
tablespoon of olive oil and mix
with some of the juice. Return it
to the pan and boil to thicken
slightly
10 Serve with boiled or steamed
new potatoes sprinkled with
rosemary.

PREPARATION TIME:
10 minutes, plus 1 hour
marinating/ COOKING TIME:
3 hours

VARIATION:
● *In Australia, kangaroo
meat is used for this dish. It is
occasionally available in UK and
is an excellent, low-fat meat.*

**IF USING A MEAT
THERMOMETER, USE
THE SETTING FOR BEEF
WHEN COOKING
VENISON.**

**VENISON IN
COCONUT MILK (10)**
This recipe was given to us by
Jeannie McKillup.

CORE INGREDIENT
1 kg venison, cut into 5 cm
cubes

FRUIT/VEGETABLES
5–6 cloves garlic
1 large onion
1 T lemon juice
4–6 spring onions, chopped

FROM THE CUPBOARD
2 cups of coconut milk
2 T olive oil

HERBS AND SPICES
salt
2 red chillies
2 tsp paprika
3–4 lime leaves
1 stalk lemon grass
2 T fresh coriander

1 Process together the olive oil,
lemon juice, garlic, onion, chillies,
paprika, lemon grass and lime
leaves to form a smooth paste
2 Add the paste to a big
saucepan or wok and fry for 2 to
3 minutes before slowly mixing
in the coconut milk
3 Add the venison and simmer
for about 1½ hours stirring
occasionally
4 Turn up the heat and
simmer strongly for another
15 minutes
5 Serve garnished with fresh
coriander and spring onions.

PREPARATION TIME:
7–8 minutes/COOKING TIME:
1 ¾ – 2 hours

7.7 DELECTABLE DESSERTS

The best dessert is a plate of
fresh fruit. Let your family
choose their favourite from a
fruit bowl or peel and cut up a
selection on individual plates or
make a fruit salad. Remember
the saying that a man will eat
an orange only if it is peeled for
him. It is certainly true in our
families! Alternatively serve a
bowl of dried fruit and nuts.

For special occasions here
is a selection of desserts most
people will enjoy.

ICE CREAM AND SORBETS

Several of the recipes contain
alcohol because of the influence
of Gill's husband David Falvey.
In almost every case this is
optional. Remember not to add
too much alcohol or your sorbet
or ice cream will not freeze!

*ICE CREAMS AND
SORBETS CAN BE MADE A
FEW HOURS BEFORE YOU
NEED THEM AND KEPT IN
THE FREEZER. LEAVE IT
TO SOFTEN IN THE
FRIDGE FOR ABOUT
15 TO 30 MINUTES
BEFORE SERVING.*

BANANA ICE CREAM (4)
CORE INGREDIENT
450 gm ripe banana, chopped

FRUIT/VEGETABLES
1 T lemon juice

FROM THE CUPBOARD
2 cups of coconut milk
3 T honey or 1/2 cup cane sugar
2 T rum (optional)

1 Blend the banana and lemon juice in a food processor until smooth
2 Heat the honey and coconut milk and stir until the honey dissolves, and then add to the banana with the rum
3 Chill and then churn in an ice cream maker.

PREPARATION TIME:
5 minutes, plus churning time

CHOCOLATE SORBET (0)
CORE INGREDIENT
1 1/2 cups of pure cocoa

FROM THE CUPBOARD
3 cups of water
1 cup of cane sugar
2 T orange or coffee liqueur
  (optional)

1 Heat the sugar and water in a saucepan and stir until the sugar dissolves

2 Add the cocoa and simmer for 15 minutes
3 Chill, stir in the liqueur and process in an ice cream maker
4 Serve with poached pears or caramelised oranges.

PREPARATION TIME:
15 minutes, plus churning time

VARIATION:
● *This is a delicous chocolate sauce that can be served with fruit or over coconut ice cream.*

COCONUT ICE-CREAM (5)
CORE INGREDIENT
3 eggs

FROM THE CUPBOARD
1/2 cup of cane sugar
400 ml coconut milk
1 T desiccated coconut
2 T rum (optional)

1 Beat the eggs and sugar together until they become pale yellow in colour
2 Slowly simmer the coconut milk with the desiccated coconut
3 Trickle the hot milk into the egg mixture beating all the time
4 Transfer to a saucepan and heat gently, beating continuously for

about 2 to 3 minutes
5 Cool, add the rum, and
process in an ice cream maker.

PREPARATION TIME:
10 minutes, plus churning time
COOKING TIME: 5 minutes

MANGO DAIQUIRI SORBET (0)

CORE INGREDIENT
500 gm fresh mango,
  skinned and deseeded

FRUIT/VEGETABLES
juice and rind of 2 small
  lemons

FROM THE CUPBOARD
3 T clear honey
1/2 cup water
2 T Bacardi and 1 T Triple Sec,
  or 3 T Cointreau (optional)

1 Dissolve the honey in the
water in a small saucepan
2 Blend all the ingredients in a
food processor, taste and add a
little more honey if necessary
3 Chill in the fridge and then
process in an ice cream maker.

PREPARATION TIME:
5 minutes, plus churning time

MANDARIN SORBET (0)
CORE INGREDIENT
1 1/2 cups of fresh mandarin juice

2 T grated mandarin skin

FRUIT/VEGETABLES
1 T lemon juice

FROM THE CUPBOARD
3 T honey or 1/2 cup of
  cane sugar
1/2 cup of Cointreau or Grand
  Marnier (optional)
1 cup of Asti Spumante or sweet
  white wine or water

1 Heat the sugar or honey
with 1/2 cup of wine or water
in a saucepan until the sugar
dissolves
2 Add to the mandarin juice,
lemon juice, remainder of wine
or water and Cointreau and stir
3 Chill well and process in an
ice cream maker.

PREPARATION TIME:
5 minutes, plus churning time

RASPBERRY SORBET (0)
CORE INGREDIENT
500 gm frozen raspberries

FRUIT/VEGETABLES
2 T lemon juice

FROM THE CUPBOARD
1/2 cup of water
3 T clear honey
2 T Kir (raspberry liqueur) or
  Cointreau (optional)

1 Heat the honey and water in a saucepan until the honey dissolves
2 Purée the raspberries in a food processor, add the sugar syrup and Kir, stir and chill in the fridge
3 Process in an ice cream maker according to the instructions.

PREPARATION TIME:
10 minutes, plus churning time

PINEAPPLE SORBET (1)
CORE INGREDIENT
1 ripe pineapple

FRUIT/VEGETABLES
juice of 1 orange

FROM THE CUPBOARD
3 T honey or 1/4 cup cane sugar
1/2 cup of water
3 T white rum (optional)

1 Boil the water and sugar to make a syrup
2 Add the peeled, cored and chopped pineapple and orange juice to the syrup and simmer for about 10 minutes
3 Cool, add the rum and purée in a food processor
4 Chill and then churn in an ice cream maker.

PREPARATION TIME: 6–7 minutes, plus churning time
COOKING TIME: 12 minutes

SUMMER FRUIT SORBET (0)
CORE INGREDIENT
500 gm frozen summer fruits

FRUIT/VEGETABLES
4 T lemon juice

FROM THE CUPBOARD
3 T honey
1/2 cup of water
1/4 cup of Campari (optional)

1 Dissolve the honey in the water in a small saucepan
2 Blend all the ingredients in a food processor, taste and add a little bit more honey if necessary
3 Chill in the fridge and then churn in an ice cream maker.

PREPARATION TIME:
5 minutes, plus churning time

SORBET SUGGESTION
● Lemon sorbet, doused in Aquavit(!)

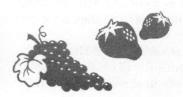

FRUIT DISHES

APPLE AND FIG CRUMBLE (3)

This recipe was given to us by Pamela Thompson.

CORE INGREDIENT
3–4 apples, cored and chopped

FRUIT/VEGETABLES
8–10 figs, chopped

FROM THE CUPBOARD
1/4 cup of water
1/4 cup of grapeseed or walnut oil
1/3 cup of dark brown sugar
1/4 cup of sesame seeds
1/2 cup of chopped walnuts
1/2 cup of oatmeal
1/2 cup of wholemeal flour

HERBS AND SPICES
1 tsp cloves
1/2 tsp cinnamon
1/2 tsp nutmeg
pinch of salt

1 Lightly poach the apples and figs with the cloves and 2 tablespoons of sugar with a little water in a covered pan for about 5 minutes or until they become soft
2 Increase heat and shake the pan until the apple becomes golden and slightly caramelised.

Put to one side
3 Mix together all the other ingredients with a fork until they form a nice 'crumble'
4 Spoon the poached apples into a baking dish, cover with the crumble topping and bake in a preheated 160°C for 30 to 40 minutes until the topping is golden
5 Serve with soya milk custard.

PREPARATION TIME:
5–6 minutes/COOKING TIME:
40–50 mins

VARIATIONS:
● Use any fruit of your choice and poach with a little sugar and water until soft.
● Add nuts, muesli and raisins to the crumble topping.

SOYA MILK CUSTARD (5)

CORE INGREDIENT
5 egg yolks

FROM THE CUPBOARD
2 cups of soya milk or 1 cup of milk and 1 cup of soya cream
1/2 cup of sugar

HERBS AND SPICES
2–3 drops vanilla essence

1 Heat the milk (and cream) with the vanilla essence until it begins to simmer

2 Whisk together the egg yolks and sugar until pale yellow and foamy, then slowly add the soya 'milk' continuing to whisk
3 Return the mixture to the pan and cook over a moderate heat, stirring constantly, until it thickens
4 Strain and serve hot or cold.

PREPARATION TIME:
5 minutes/COOKING TIME:
10 minutes

VARIATION:
● *To make this into ice-cream, add 2 tablespoons of Grand Marnier (optional), cool the mixture and process in an ice cream maker.*

FRUIT PIES
● *STEP 1 – PASTRY*
CORE INGREDIENT
1 egg, separated

FROM THE CUPBOARD
240 gm plain flour
60 gm softened solid vegetable
  oil, cut into small cubes
2–3 T water

HERBS AND SPICES
pinch of salt

1 Add all the ingredients, except the egg white, to a food processor and process until it forms a firm dough. Adjust the water or flour as necessary. Knead the dough slightly, wrap it in a tea towel and cool it in the fridge for 30 minutes
2 Preheat the oven to 200°C
3 Dust the pastry with flour and roll it out as thinly as possible. Roll it over a rolling pin and fit it into the pie tin
4 Press it into the edges of the tin and trim, leaving some pastry overhanging because it will shrink while cooking. Prick the base and brush it with the egg white
5 Bake in a preheated 200°C oven for about 20 minutes until it becomes slightly golden.

PREPARATION TIME:
5 minutes, plus 30 minutes in the fridge/COOKING TIME:
20 minutes

SHORT CUT: You can buy shortcrust pastry which does not contain dairy.

● *STEP 2 – LEMON FILLING (8)*
CORE INGREDIENT
6 small eggs

FRUIT/VEGETABLES
zest and juice of 6 large lemons

FROM THE CUPBOARD
175 gm cane sugar
200 ml soya 'cream'

1 Beat together the eggs and sugar until they become pale yellow and form ribbons
2 Add the lemon juice and zest and stir well
3 Whisk in the soya 'cream'
4 Pour into the just-cooked pastry case and bake in a 160°C oven for 30 to 40 minutes until almost set
5 Allow to cool before serving.

PREPARATION TIME:
10 minutes/COOKING TIME:
30–40 minutes

VARIATION:
● *Apple with apricot purée (spread apricot purée over the warm pastry to form a base and cover with overlapping sliced apples)*

PIE SUGGESTIONS
● Almond paste and figs.
● Custard tart
● Poached apricots with pine nuts.
● Fresh strawberry with raspberry purée and cold egg custard base (not cooked).

POACHED CHERRIES (3)
CORE INGREDIENT
500 gm black cherries

FRUIT/VEGETABLES
2 T lemon juice

FROM THE CUPBOARD
1/2 cup cane sugar
1 T kirsch

1 Put the cherries in a pan with the sugar and lemon juice, cover and simmer gently for about 10 minutes
2 Remove the fruit and boil the remaining liquid rapidly until it reduces then add the kirsch
3 Pour the sauce over the cherries and serve immediately.

PREPARATION TIME:
1 minute/COOKING TIME:
5–6 minutes

MARINATED ORANGES (0)
CORE INGREDIENT
5 oranges

FRUIT/VEGETABLES
2 T lemon juice

FROM THE CUPBOARD
2–3 T sugar
2 T Cointreau or Grand Marnier (optional)

1 Peel four of the oranges, cut them into thick slices, then in half and place them in a flat wide bowl. Juice the remaining oranges
2 Sprinkle with sugar and pour over the orange and lemon juice and Cointreau

3 Leave the oranges to marinate for at least two hours, but preferably overnight, turning the slices occasionally.

PREPARATION TIME:
5 minutes, plus 2 hours minimum marinating

POACHED PEARS (3)
CORE INGREDIENT
4 pears, peeled

FRUIT/VEGETABLES
1 cm fresh ginger, slivered
grated lemon rind

FROM THE
CUPBOARD
1 cup cane sugar
4 cups of water

HERBS AND
SPICES
1 vanilla pod

1 Place all the ingredients in a saucepan and simmer, turning the pears occasionally, for about 30 minutes or until they are soft
2 Drain the pears and serve with a little of the syrup in which they have been cooked.

PREPARATION TIME:
5 minutes/COOKING TIME:
30 minutes

ROAST FRUIT (3)
CORE INGREDIENT
2 peaches, quartered and the stone removed

FRUIT/VEGETABLES
4 plums, halved and stone
  removed
2 nectarines, quartered and
  deseeded
4 apricots, halved
2 punnets blueberries

FROM THE CUPBOARD
1/2 cup of Amaretto or a sweet
  wine or sherry
1/2 cup of toasted almonds
2 T brown sugar

1 Toast the almonds in a dry pan until they change colour
2 Put all the fruit in a baking tray
3 Mix together the Amaretto and sugar and pour over the fruit
4 Bake in a preheated 180°C oven for about 15 minutes until the fruit is soft
5 Stir in the blueberries just before serving and sprinkle with toasted almonds
6 Serve with coconut ice cream (4) and/or almond macaroons (5).

PREPARATION TIME:
10 minutes/COOKING TIME:
17–18 minutes

SPICED APRICOTS WITH TOASTED ALMONDS (3)

CORE INGREDIENT
3–4 apricots per person

FROM THE CUPBOARD
1/4 cup of sugar
1/3 cup of water
1/2 cup of sweet dessert wine
 or sherry (optional)
1/2 cup of almond slivers

HERBS AND SPICES
1 vanilla pod or 3–4 drops
vanilla essence

1 Toast the almonds briefly in the oven or in a dry pan until they change colour
2 Boil the water and sugar together and stir until the sugar dissolves. Add the wine and vanilla and simmer for 5 minutes
3 Cut the apricots into quarters and remove the kernel, add the apricots to the syrup and simmer for 3 to 4 minutes until the apricots are soft
4 Stir in the almonds just before serving.

PREPARATION TIME:
5 minutes/COOKING TIME:
10 minutes

SUMMER PUDDING (3)

This is a classic dish.

CORE INGREDIENT
500 gm frozen summer fruits
 (thawed)

FRUIT/VEGETABLES
1 punnet raspberries
1 punnet redcurrants
 (if available)

FROM THE CUPBOARD
thinly sliced white bread,
 crusts removed
1/2 cup of cane sugar
1/2 cup of water

1 Heat the sugar and water and stir until the sugar has dissolved
2 Add the frozen fruit, with their juice, the raspberries and redcurrants, stir, cover and bring to a boil for 1 to 2 minutes
3 Remove from the heat and leave to cool
4 Strain the fruit reserving the liquid
5 Line a 1 litre-capacity basin with the bread, cutting it to fit; do not leave gaps
6 Tip the fruit into the bread and pour over some of the reserved juice, then cover the top with bread
7 Cover the pudding with foil, then top with a saucer that just fits inside the basin and weigh it

down with some heavy objects and leave it at least overnight

8 To serve, remove the weights, saucer and foil, place a serving dish underneath and carefully invert the pudding

9 The pudding should be bright crimson in colour; if there are gaps in the colour just pour over some of the reserved liquid

10 Serve with extra juice and nut paste.

PREPARATION TIME:
10–15 minutes, plus overnight marinating/COOKING TIME:
2–3 minutes

NUT PASTE (1)
FROM THE CUPBOARD
1 cup of unsalted cashew nuts
1/4 –1/2 cup of water

HERBS AND SPICES
2–3 drops vanilla essence

1 Blend the cashew nuts, vanilla essence and water together in a food processor, slowly adding water until the mixture forms a smooth 'creamy' texture.

PREPARATION TIME: 2–3 mins

TROPICAL FRUIT WITH GINGER WINE (0)
CORE INGREDIENT
1 small pineapple

FRUIT/VEGETABLES
2 oranges
1 mango
2 kiwi fruit
2 passion fruit
1/2 tsp fresh ginger, grated
grated rind from 1 small lemon

FROM THE CUPBOARD
3 T ginger wine
1 T slivered almonds, toasted

1 Toast the almonds in a small pan for a few minutes until they change colour

2 Peel, core and slice the pineapple, orange, mango and kiwifruit and mix together gently in a serving bowl. Squeeze the seeds of the passion fruit over the other fruit

3 Warm the ginger wine with the fresh ginger and grated lemon rind in a small saucepan and pour it over the fruit and garnish with the toasted almonds

4 Serve with coconut ice cream or meringues (5).

PREPARATION TIME:
10–15 minutes/COOKING TIME: 1–2 minutes

MERINGUES (8)
CORE INGREDIENT
1 egg white

FROM THE CUPBOARD
3/4 cup of cane sugar
3 T water
1 tsp lemon juice
2 tsp cornflour

1 Heat the sugar and water together stirring continuously until the sugar dissolves and bring to the boil
2 Beat the egg white until it becomes stiff
3 Add the lemon juice and cornflour while still beating
4 Slowly add the boiling syrup to the egg and continue to beat until the mixture is thick and holds its shape
5 Put the mixture into a piping bag and pipe meringues on to foil on a baking tray
6 Bake in a very slow oven for about 40 minutes until the meringue is firm and dry
7 Cool in the oven with the door ajar.

PREPARATION TIME:
10 minutes/COOKING TIME:
40 minutes

FRUIT SALAD SUGGESTIONS
● Orange, melon and passion fruit (0)
● Pineapple, strawberries, banana, apple and passion fruit (0)

OTHER DESSERTS

COCONUT CRÊPES WITH APRICOT PURÉE(5)
CORE INGREDIENT
3 eggs

FROM THE CUPBOARD
1 1/2 cups of plain flour
3 cups of coconut milk
soya spread for frying crêpes

HERBS AND SPICES
2 tsp salt

1 Sift the flour and salt into a bowl and add the coconut milk, slowly mixing with a whisk
2 Lightly beat the eggs and add to the batter, whisking the mixture until it is smooth
3 Heat a little soya spread in a frying pan, add a ladle of the mixture and cook until the underside turns a golden brown, flip the pancake and cook the other side
4 Serve with apricot purée.

This makes 10 to 12 crêpes about 20 cm across.

PREPARATION TIME:
5–6 minutes/COOKING TIME:
1–2 minutes per crêpe

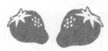

VARIATION:
● *Spread with lemon and honey, or maple syrup or with caramelised oranges and orange syrup.*

COCONUT CRÈME CARAMEL (5)
CORE INGREDIENT
3 medium eggs

FROM THE CUPBOARD
1 cup cane sugar
1 cup coconut milk
1/2 cup water

HERBS AND SPICES
1 tsp vanilla essence

1 Put the sugar and water in a saucepan and heat gently stirring until the sugar is dissolved, then boil rapidly until the liquid turns golden brown
2 Pour the sugar syrup into a 500ml ovenproof dish or individual ramekin dishes
3 Whisk together the coconut milk and eggs and pour the mixture into the ovenproof dish or ramekins on top of the caramelised sugar
4 Place the dish or dishes in a baking tray containing about 1/2 inch of water and bake in the oven preheated to 160°C for about 45 minutes or until the custards feel firm to the touch

5 Refrigerate and serve cold by carefully inverting the dish or ramekins on to the serving dishes. The custard should be surrounded by dark caramel
6 Serve by itself or with marinated oranges (page 207–8).

PREPARATION TIME:
5–6 minutes/COOKING TIME:
50–55 minutes

COCONUT AND GINGER CRÈME BRULÉE (5)
CORE INGREDIENT
3 eggs

FROM THE CUPBOARD
1 cup coconut milk
1/2 cup preserved ginger syrup
5–6 pieces preserved ginger
4 T dark brown sugar

1 Purée the ginger and syrup in a blender or food processor
2 Beat the eggs slightly and add to the ginger syrup
3 Add the coconut milk and blend together
4 Pour the mixture into a saucepan and cook over a low heat until the mixture coats the back of a spoon
5 Pour into individual soufflé dishes, cover and refrigerate overnight
6 To serve, sprinkle dark brown sugar over each crème and heat

under the grill until the sugar caramelises. Alternatively, when cool, sprinkle with sugar and return to the fridge.

PREPARATION TIME:
5–6 minutes/COOKING TIME:
20–30 minutes

COCONUT GRAPE BRULÉE (5)
CORE INGREDIENT
3 eggs

FRUIT/VEGETABLES
2 cups seedless red and green grapes, halved

FROM THE CUPBOARD
1 cup coconut milk
1/2 cup cane sugar
4 T brown sugar

HERBS AND SPICES
1 T ground ginger

1 Lightly beat the eggs and sugar until they become pale yellow in colour
2 Heat the coconut milk and ground ginger to a slow simmer, then add it slowly to the egg mixture
3 Return the mixture to the saucepan and heat gently until it coats the back of a spoon
4 Put the grapes in a serving dish, spoon over the coconut

custard and leave it in the refrigerator overnight
5 Before serving, sprinkle the brown sugar over the custard and place under a hot grill for 3 to 4 minutes until the sugar caramelises. Alternatively, when the custards are cool, sprinkle with sugar and return to the fridge.

PREPARATION TIME:
5–6 minutes/COOKING TIME:
20–30 minutes

VARIATION:
● *Use raspberries or blueberries instead of the grapes.*

ORANGE AND ALMOND CUSTARDS (5)
CORE INGREDIENT
1 egg plus 3 egg yolks

FRUIT/VEGETABLES
1 cup of orange juice
  (2–3 oranges)

FROM THE CUPBOARD
3 T clear honey
1/2 cup of water
2 T ground almonds
2 T pistachio nuts,
  coarsely ground
2 T Cointreau or
  Grand Marnier
  (optional)

1 Heat the honey and water and stir until the honey has dissolved

2 Add the orange juice and simmer for 2 to 3 minutes until it thickens slightly then leave it to cool

3 Beat the eggs until they are pale and creamy, and slowly add the orange syrup, beating continuously

4 Add the ground almonds and the Cointreau and mix well

5 Pour into a soufflé dish or individual dishes placed in a baking tray half filled with water and bake in a preheated 180°C oven for about 40 minutes until set

6 Serve sprinkled with chopped pistachio nuts.

PREPARATION TIME:
10 minutes/COOKING TIME:
40–45 mins

RICE PUDDING WITH PALM SUGAR AND COCONUT MILK (4)
CORE INGREDIENT
1 cup of short grained rice

FROM THE CUPBOARD
2 cups of coconut milk
2 cups of water
1 cup palm sugar or
  brown sugar

1 Heat the palm sugar with half a cup of water to form a thick syrup, stirring until the sugar dissolves

2 Put the rice, two tablespoons of the sugar syrup, one cup of coconut milk and one and a half cups of water into a saucepan and simmer gently, until the rice is cooked. If the liquid dries up before the rice is cooked add more water

3 Put into individual dishes and cool

4 Turn out on to plates and serve with extra palm sugar syrup and chilled coconut milk

5 This dish is especially delicious after a hot curry.

PREPARATION TIME:
2–3 minutes/COOKING TIME:
20–30 mins

VARIATION:
● *Traditionally this is made with sago or tapioca.*

CAKES

BANANA BREAD (5)
CORE INGREDIENT
2 large eggs separated

FRUIT/VEGETABLES
100 ml orange juice
2 medium ripe bananas

FROM THE CUPBOARD
300 gm plain flour
1 tsp bicarbonate of soda
1 tsp mixed spice
1 tsp ground ginger
60 gm light soft brown sugar
4 T clear honey

HERBS AND SPICES
salt

1 Sift the flour and salt into a
bowl and add the sugar
2 In a separate bowl mash the
bananas to a pulp, add the egg
yolks, honey and orange juice
and mix well
3 In a third bowl beat the egg
whites until they form soft
peaks
4 Stir the banana mixture
through the dry ingredients
until it is thoroughly mixed,
then gently fold in the egg
whites
5 Pour the mixture into a tin
and bake in a preheated 160°C
oven for 1 to 1½ hours
6 Allow the cake to cool before
turning it out of the tin. It is
better if left for a day before
eating.

Use a loaf tin 16 x 9 x 8 cm

PREPARATION TIME:
10–15 minutes/COOKING
TIME: 1–1½ hours

CARROT CAKE (5)
CORE INGREDIENT
2 eggs

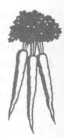

FRUIT/VEGETABLES
2 cups of finely grated
carrot (4–5)

FROM THE CUPBOARD
125 gm self-raising flour
¼ cup of dark brown
muscavado sugar
⅔ cup of olive oil
½ cup of roughly chopped
walnuts
½ cup of sultanas

HERBS AND SPICES
½ tsp ground cinnamon
½ tsp ground nutmeg
½ tsp ground ginger

1 Preheat the oven to 180°C
2 Mix together the flour, sugar
and spices in a food processor,
add the olive oil and eggs and
process for 1 minute, then stir
in the carrots and walnuts
3 Pour the mixture into an 18
cm springform tin and bake
for about 1 hour
4 Cool the cake in the tin
before turning it out.

PREPARATION TIME:
5 minutes/COOKING TIME:
60 minutes

CHOCOLATE AND APRICOT PAN FORTE (2)
CORE INGREDIENT
180 gm dark chocolate, melted

FROM THE CUPBOARD
1 cup of liquid glucose
3/4 cup of cane sugar
2 cups of almonds
1 1/2 cups of dried apricots
  and dates
1 1/2 cups of plain flour
1/3 cup of cocoa

HERBS AND SPICES
1 tsp ground cinnamon

1 Toast the almonds and
coarsely chop them in a food
processor
2 Chop the dried apricots and
dates
3 Heat the glucose syrup and
sugar in a pan and stir until the
sugar dissolves, bring to a boil
and simmer for 2 to 3 minutes
until the syrup thickens slightly
4 Mix together the almonds,
apricots, dates, flour, cocoa and
cinnamon in a bowl and add the
syrup and melted chocolate
5 Press into a greased baking tin
and cook in a preheated 180°C
oven for 20 minutes
6 Leave the cake to cool and
cut into squares.

PREPARATION TIME:
10 minutes/COOKING TIME:
20 minutes

CHOCOLATE CAKE (8)
This recipe was contributed
by Kate Lowe.

CORE INGREDIENT
4 medium eggs

FROM THE CUPBOARD
120 gm muscovado sugar
200 gm dark chocolate (at least
  70% cocoa solids)
1 T plain flour
150 gm vegetable shortening,
  or 1/3 cup of grapeseed oil
2 T cocoa powder
1/2 cup of water
2 T brandy (optional)

1 Add the cocoa powder and
water to a saucepan, bring to the
boil and stir to mix well
2 Add the vegetable shortening
or oil, chocolate and sugar and
stir until well mixed
3 Beat the eggs lightly and add
slowly to the chocolate whisking
continuously
4 Add the flour continuing to
whisk ensuring there are no
lumps, then stir in the brandy
5 Pour into a greased 20 cm
cake tin and bake in an oven
preheated to 180°C for 30
minutes

6 Leave the cake to cool in the cake tin then put in a container and chill in the fridge for a few hours before serving.

PREPARATION TIME:
10 minutes/COOKING TIME:
30 mins

HAZELNUT, CHOCOLATE AND DATE MERINGUE CAKE (5)

Gill's stepdaughter, Kate Gibbons, contributed this recipe for a sophisticated dinner party dessert.

CORE INGREDIENT
6 egg whites

FRUIT/VEGETABLES
250 gm seedless dates

FROM THE CUPBOARD
100 gm chopped almonds
100 gm chopped hazelnuts
250 gm Belgian dark chocolate
125 gm cane sugar

HERBS AND SPICES
1/2 tsp salt

1 Break the chocolate into pieces and add it to a food processor and process until it is coarsely chopped
2 Chop the dates as finely as possible
3 Beat the egg whites with the salt until they form stiff peaks, then gradually add the sugar and beat until stiff
4 Add the almonds, hazelnuts, chocolate and dates to the eggs and fold in gently
5 Grease the base of a springform pan or use a piece of greased foil or greaseproof paper, pour in the mixture and bake in an oven preheated to 160°C for about 45 minutes. Allow the torte to cool in the oven with the door open
6 Refrigerate for at least 6 hours before serving
7 Serve cold with mixed berries and soya or nut 'cream'.

PREPARATION TIME:
15 minutes, plus 6 hours resting/ COOKING TIME:
45 minutes

ORANGE AND ALMOND CAKE (8)

This is a classic Middle Eastern cake that Diana Lampe introduced to us. The taste depends on the quality of the oranges used. Select thin-skinned ripe sweet oranges.

CORE INGREDIENT
4 medium eggs

FRUIT/VEGETABLES
2 medium oranges
1 small lemon

FROM THE CUPBOARD
200 gm ground almonds
250 gm cane sugar
1 tsp baking powder

1 Boil the oranges in a covered saucepan in a little water for 2 hours, add the lemon after 1 hour and add extra water if the pan goes dry

2 Allow the oranges and lemon to cool, chop them coarsely and remove any pips and add to the food processor with the ground almonds, sugar and baking powder and process until mixed thoroughly

3 Add the eggs and continue to process until smooth

4 Pour into a greased and floured springform tin and bake in a preheated 180°C oven for about an hour. If it is still very wet continue to cook a little longer

5 Cool the cake in the tin before turning it out

6 Serve with soya 'cream' and caramelised oranges.

PREPARATION TIME:
5 minutes/COOKING TIME:
2 hours for the oranges and lemon, plus 1 hour baking

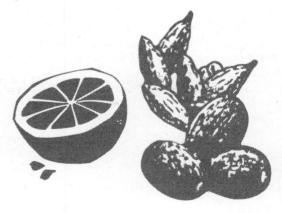

8 Feeding the family

8.1 KIDS' STUFF

Teaching children how to eat properly is one of the most important lessons you can give them. Good nutrition in childhood can be the foundation of lifelong good health. Bad eating habits in childhood can lead to cancer and heart attacks in later life. Also, many childhood ailments such as eczema, asthma and catarrh can be cleared up, or at least helped by simply removing dairy produce and cutting down on junk food.

To engage children in cooking and good eating, it is important to make meals and snacks *fun*. Never be uptight about food, because many children will learn to use not eating as a means of gaining attention. Ensure kids do not eat sweets or chocolates between meals, or have sweet fruity drinks with their meals (the instant high blood sugar will kill their appetite). Use packets of raisins, or dried fruit as treats and snacks.

Small children can be tempted to eat food that is cut into attractive shapes. Buy pastry cutters and turn breaded fish fillets into 'baby fish' shapes. Stamp out alphabet, or other shapes from toast or mashed potatoes. Make potato faces with baked potatoes, using beans for eyes, a cherry tomato or tiny carrot for a nose, and a slice of red pepper for the mouth. Fruit can be treated in a similar way, creating apple, pear or peach faces. However, be warned that a small minority of children will want to keep the potato or fruit faces, or baby fish, rather than eat them!

TIPS FOR YOUNGER CHILDREN:
- *CUT UP VEGETABLES VERY SMALL OR PURÉE*
- *GIVE AN EXOTIC FRUIT AS A TREAT – BUT IN THE AFTERNOON, RATHER THAN THE MORNING*
- *ENCOURAGE KIDS TO 'JUST TRY IT'*
- *GIVE DRIED FRUITS (BUT NOT NUTS) AS SNACKS*
- *INVOLVE THE KIDS IN YOUR COOKING AND GIVE THEM ALL TASKS TO DO – THEY WILL LEARN HOW TO COOK AND YOU WILL FEEL MORE RELAXED.*

8.2 TEENS TO TWENTIES

Teenagers are often the most difficult people to feed, because they are trying to establish a separate identity, independent of that which they had as their parents' children. They may decide suddenly to become vegetarian, or to rebel against the food their parents have always encouraged them to eat. In these situations parental pressure to conform can be quite counterproductive.

One of the best techniques for encouraging teenagers to eat well is to leave information around for them to read for themselves (without comment). For example, buy magazines suitable for their age group, which give good sound advice. Also, leave *this* book around for them to explore. It is designed to appeal to young people and the Virgin logo might tempt them to open it. Work with them as their sous chef, to develop healthy and nutritious meals that they can enjoy. Encourage them to give supper parties for their peers, and help them to cook the food.

Most teenagers are desperate to look good and if you can help them to understand the connection between looking good and eating well they will be more likely to adopt a healthier diet. For example, many youngsters suffer badly from acne during their teens. This can frequently be cleared up by eliminating dairy and junk food, cutting back on meat, and increasing the proportion of fresh fruit and vegetables that they eat.

Teenagers have school pressures and busy social lives, so they have little spare time for cooking. All the recipes in this book are healthy, tasty and nutritious, and as our children were growing up, they have eaten and enjoyed many of them. Here are some suggestions to get you and your children started.

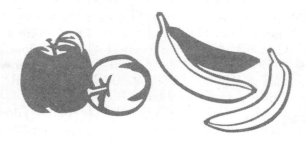

FRUITY THINGS

BANANA WHIP (0)
CORE INGREDIENT
4 bananas

FROM THE CUPBOARD
honey to taste

1 Wrap peeled bananas in foil and freeze
2 Chop coarsely and process the frozen bananas in a food processor until they become thick and creamy. Add honey to taste.
Serve in a special dish, or in an ice cream cone.

PREPARATION TIME:
1–2 minutes, plus freezing time

APPLE AND SUGAR SANDWICHES (3)
CORE INGREDIENT
1 green apple

FRUIT/VEGETABLES
1 tsp lemon juice

FROM THE CUPBOARD
raw cane sugar to taste
2 slices fresh bread

1 Peel, core and slice the apple, and toss in lemon juice to stop it going brown
2 Put the apple slices on the bread, sprinkle with sugar and top with another slice of bread.

Our children used to like really sour cooking apples for these sandwiches.

PREPARATION TIME:
2–3 minutes

APPLE FRITTERS (3)
CORE INGREDIENT
2–3 Granny Smith apples

FRUIT/VEGETABLES
1 T lemon juice

FROM THE CUPBOARD
1/2 cup water
1/2 cup wholemeal flour
unrefined cane sugar to taste
grapeseed or sunflower oil for
    shallow frying

1 Peel, core and slice the apples and toss in lemon juice to stop them going brown
2 To make the batter, add water to a soup plate and then gradually add the flour, sifting it through a sieve/shaker and beating continuously with a fork. Adjust water and flour as necessary to make a batter with the consistency of medium 'cream'
3 Add about 1/2 cm (1/4") depth of oil to a frying pan and heat.

When the oil is quite hot, dip the apple in the batter, add to the pan and cook until a fine golden crust forms on one side; then turn over the fritter and do the other side
4 Serve sprinkled with sugar to taste.

PREPARATION TIME:
2–3 minutes/COOKING TIME:
5 minutes

VARIATION:
● *Add cinnamon powder to the flour or sugar*

BANANA ON TOAST/ BANANA SANDWICH (3)
CORE INGREDIENT
1 banana

FROM THE CUPBOARD
2 slices fresh bread
1 tsp honey or raw cane sugar
1 tsp soya 'milk' or cream

1 Mash the banana with the honey or sugar and soya 'milk' or cream and pile on top of one slice of bread. Top with the other to make a sandwich.

PREPARATION TIME:
1–2 minutes

SHAKES AND SMOOTHIES

Rich fruit smoothies, or soya 'milk' shakes are a good way to get your children to enjoy drinks that are healthier than the bottled sweetened commercial versions. They are made simply by blending soft fruit in a blender with soya 'milk' and a spoonful of honey to taste.

BANANA AND SOYA 'MILK' SHAKE (1)
CORE INGREDIENT
1 banana

FROM THE CUPBOARD
1 cup soya 'milk'
1 T honey or to taste

1 Purée the banana, soya 'milk' and honey in the food processor until smooth.

PREPARATION TIME:
1–2 minutes

Soft fruits such as bananas, peaches, nectarines, apricots, papaya and strawberries form the basis of wonderful smoothies/shakes. These fruits can be frozen before blending to make an ice cold dessert.

OTHER SMOOTHIE IDEAS

● Blend 1/2 banana with 1/2 cup strawberries and the juice from 2 oranges (0)
● Blend 1 peach with 1 banana and the juice from 1 orange (0)
● Blend 1 cup of strawberries with the juice from 2 pears (0)

RASPBERRIES OR APRICOTS WITH FRENCH TOAST (5)

This is also known as 'eggy bread'. If you are concerned about giving kids beer bread, don't be! By the time the dough has been in the oven for 40 to 45 minutes, at 220°C, there will be no alcohol left in the loaf. The beer is for flavour, not intoxication. However, you can use any bread you like, as long as it does not contain dairy.

CORE INGREDIENT
2 eggs

FRUIT/VEGETABLES
raspberries or apricots

FROM THE CUPBOARD
4 slices of beer bread (from the breakfast section)
1/2 cup of soya 'milk'
1/4 tsp salt
soya spread for frying

HERBS AND SPICES
cinnamon powder
sugar to taste

1 Cut 4 slices of bread, about 1 cm thick, mix the sugar and cinnamon to taste on a plate
2 Whisk the eggs, add the salt and soya 'milk' and pour into a shallow bowl
3 Soak 2 slices of bread at a time in the egg mixture, for a minute or so, turning to coat both sides of the bread
4 Warm a little soya butter in a frying pan to coat the bottom of the pan, and fry the 'eggy bread' in a medium hot, non-stick pan, until both sides are medium brown
5 Dip into sugar/cinnamon mix, serve hot with raspberries or apricots on the side.

PREPARATION TIME:
5 minutes/COOKING TIME:
5 minutes

STRAWBERRIES WITH SOYA 'MILK' PANCAKES (5)

The same arguments about kids and beer batters put under 'French toast' apply to these pancakes. It is all about flavour, and the juxtaposition of bitterness and sweetness (just like living with teenagers, really).

CORE INGREDIENT
1 egg

FRUIT/VEGETABLES
1 cup soya 'milk'
1 cup beer
100 gm strawberries
lemon juice to taste

FROM THE CUPBOARD
220 gm plain flour
soya spread to cook individual
    pancakes
raw cane sugar to taste

HERBS AND SPICES
1 tsp salt

1 Mix the flour, sugar and salt in a bowl, add the soya 'milk' and beer and whisk
2 Add the egg and continue to whisk to a smooth batter
3 Put a little soya 'butter' into a hot frying pan, pour up to about 100 ml of batter into the pan and run it around to make a thin pancake that covers the base of the pan
4 Cook for about one minute and then flip to cook the other side
5 Serve on to a plate, add sliced strawberries, sprinkle with sugar to taste, drizzle over lemon juice and roll.

These quantities will make about 500 ml of batter; enough for 5 large, or 6 to 7 small pancakes.

PREPARATION TIME:
5 minutes/COOKING TIME:
5 minutes

VARIATION:
● *These pancakes can be served with an infinite variety of fillings. Fruit, banana with chocolate sauce, or even chocolate sauce on its own, maple syrup, apricot purée and sorbets are all delicious.*

DESSERTS AND SNACKS

CHOCOLATE 'MILK' (1)
CORE INGREDIENT
50 gm dark, dairy-free chocolate, diced

FROM THE CUPBOARD
1 cup soya 'milk'
sugar to taste

1 Heat the soya 'milk'
2 Put the diced chocolate into a glass or mug and pour over the hot soya 'milk'. Stir until the chocolate is melted. Add sugar to taste.

PREPARATION TIME: 1 minute
COOKING TIME: 5 minutes

VARIATION:
● *Use 100% cocoa powder instead of chocolate.*

PEANUT BUTTER BISCUITS (8)

Another recipe contributed by Jeannie McKillop.

CORE INGREDIENT
1 cup coarse peanut butter

FROM THE CUPBOARD
1/2 cup honey
1/2 cup sesame oil
2 cups plain flour

HERBS AND SPICES
1/2 tsp vanilla essence
1/2 tsp salt

1 Mix together the peanut butter, honey, oil, salt and vanilla essence until smooth
2 Add the flour and mix well to form a dough
3 Divide into small balls, flatten into a biscuit shape and place on a greased baking tray
4 Bake in an oven preheated to 180°C for about 10 minutes, watching carefully to ensure they do not burn.

This mixture should make 25–30 biscuits.

PREPARATION TIME:
10–15 minutes/COOKING TIME: 10 minutes

PECAN BISCUITS (8)

CORE INGREDIENT
3 egg whites

FROM THE CUPBOARD
1 cup pecan nuts
1 cup brown sugar

HERBS AND SPICES
1 tsp vanilla essence

1 Add the nuts to a food processor and process until finely ground
2 Beat the egg whites until they form stiff peaks, then gradually add the sugar, while still beating until it again forms stiff peaks. Gently fold in the nuts and vanilla
3 Put teaspoonfuls of the mixture on a greased and floured baking tray, and bake for about 10 to 15 minutes in a preheated 180°C oven. Cool on a wire rack.

The mixture should make about 20 biscuits.

PREPARATION TIME:
10 minutes/COOKING TIME: 15 minutes

COCONUT MILK RICE PUDDING (4)
CORE INGREDIENT
1 cup short grain rice

FROM THE CUPBOARD
2 1/2 cups coconut milk
1 cup water
1/2 cup cane sugar

HERBS AND SPICES
1/2 tsp cinnamon or nutmeg
2 cloves

1 Put the rice in a large pan, sprinkle over the sugar, pour over the coconut milk and water
2 Sprinkle with the cinnamon or nutmeg, add the cloves and put in a preheated 180°C oven and bake for about an hour.

Serve with poached fruits (3).

PREPARATION TIME:
1 minute/COOKING TIME:
60 minutes

VARIATION:
● *This can be made on top of the stove, just stir regularly to avoid it sticking to the pan.*

APRICOT BALLS (1)
CORE INGREDIENT
3/4 cup of dried apricots and seedless dates

FRUIT/VEGETABLES
1 tsp orange peel
1 tsp lemon peel
1 T fresh orange juice

FROM THE CUPBOARD
3/4 cup of desiccated coconut
extra coconut

1 Pour boiling water over the apricots and dates and leave to soak for 10 minutes, then drain and finely chop
2 Add the coconut, lemon and orange rinds, and fresh orange juice and mix well (if the mixture is too dry add some more orange juice, if it is too wet add some more coconut)
3 Shape into small balls, roll in the extra coconut and refrigerate for at least 30 minutes

PREPARATION TIME:
15 minutes, plus 30 minutes for chilling

COCONUT BALLS (5)
CORE INGREDIENT
1 large egg

FROM THE CUPBOARD
2 1/2 cups of desiccated coconut
3/4 cup of cane sugar
2 T self-raising flour
1/4 cup of soya 'milk'

HERBS AND SPICES
2-3 drops vanilla essence

1 Mix the coconut, sugar and flour together
2 Lightly beat the egg, soya 'milk' and vanilla
3 Pour the egg mixture on to the desiccated coconut and mix together well
4 Roll into small balls, pressing together firmly
5 Place on a baking tray on top of foil and bake in a preheated 160°C oven for about 25-30 minutes until they are golden brown.

PREPARATION TIME:
10-15 minutes/COOKING TIME: 25-30 minutes

COCONUT TOFFEE (1)
CORE INGREDIENT
1 cup desiccated coconut

FROM THE CUPBOARD
1 cup raw cane sugar
1/2 cup water
1 tsp white vinegar

1 Heat the water, sugar and vinegar in a saucepan and stir until the sugar dissolves
2 Boil for 5 to 7 minutes until the liquid is golden in colour (it should solidify when a teaspoonful is dropped in a little cold water)
3 Pour into a greased flat pan and leave to cool
4 Break into pieces.

PREPARATION TIME:
5-7 minutes, plus 30 minutes cooling time/COOKING TIME: 6-8 minutes

SAVOURY DISHES

CHICKEN BURGERS (9)
The 'ingredients' in these chicken burgers will be determined by what your child will eat, so if he or she doesn't like garlic or peas or onions, just miss them out. If making them for adults, add one fresh red chilli and some chopped parsley or coriander.
CORE INGREDIENT
4-6 deboned and skinned chicken thighs, minced

FRUIT/VEGETABLES
3 spring onions, chopped
1 T ginger, minced
1-2 cloves garlic, minced (optional)
1/4 cup of peas, thawed if using frozen peas

FROM THE CUPBOARD
1 T sesame oil
1 T light soya sauce
2 T roasted sesame seeds

HERBS AND SPICES
salt and pepper to taste

1 Heat a non-stick frying pan, add the sesame seeds and toast for about 1 to 2 minutes whilst tossing them around
2 Add all the ingredients to the chicken mince and mix well
3 Heat a griddle pan, divide the chicken mixture into individual 'burgers' and add to the pan
4 Cook for about 2 minutes on one side until the 'burgers' turn brown, then turn them over and brown the other side. Turn the heat to medium low and cook, keep turning the 'burgers' until they are cooked through, about 6 minutes for each side in total.

PREPARATION TIME:
10 minutes/COOKING TIME: 15 minutes

VARIATION:
● *If making these for adults, or children who will eat chilli, add 1 to 2 red chillies and fry with the garlic and ginger.*

TO TOAST SESAME SEEDS, ADD TO A HOT DRY PAN AND KEEP TOSSING. TO AVOID BURNING THEM TURN OFF THE HEAT AFTER ABOUT A MINUTE AS THEY WILL CONTINUE TO COOK IN THE HOT PAN.

FISH FINGERS (9)
CORE INGREDIENT
300 gm firm white skinless and boneless fish
1 medium egg yolk

FROM THE CUPBOARD
3 slices day-old white bread with crusts removed
1 T plain flour
3–4 T sunflower oil

HERBS AND SPICES
salt and black pepper to taste

1 Cut the fish widthways into even 'fish fingers'
2 Process the bread in a food processor to make fine breadcrumbs, then tip them out on to a flat plate
3 Put the flour on to another plate and season to taste with salt and pepper
4 Lightly beat the egg in a bowl big enough to fit one fish finger
5 Dip the fish fingers first in the flour, then in the egg, and then

the breadcrumbs
6 Heat the oil in a frying pan or wok, and shallow fry for 2–3 minutes each side until just cooked
7 Drain on kitchen paper before serving garnished with a little parsley.

PREPARATION TIME:
10 minutes/COOKING TIME:
5–6 minutes

POTATO WEDGES (3)
CORE INGREDIENT
4 medium potatoes, cut into large wedges

FRUIT/VEGETABLES
2 cloves garlic, minced (optional)

FROM THE CUPBOARD
2 T olive oil

HERBS AND SPICES
1 tsp paprika
salt to taste

1 Dry the potatoes in kitchen paper and put them into a bowl
2 Pour over the oil, garlic, paprika, salt and pepper, and mix well ensuring that the potatoes are covered in the oil
3 Arrange the potatoes in a single layer on a greased baking tray

4 Bake in a preheated 210°C oven for about 20 minutes.

PREPARATION TIME:
5 minutes/COOKING TIME:
20 minutes

VARIATION:
● *Sweet potato with cumin.*

PIZZA (3)
Gill's stepson, Patrick Falvey, tested and contributed this recipe for a really moreish, non-dairy pizza, which he and his 'beer-swilling mates' really love.

STAGE 1
CORE INGREDIENT
700 gm strong plain white flour

FROM THE CUPBOARD
14 gm instant dried yeast
pinch of sugar
500 ml warm water
4 T olive oil

HERBS AND SPICES
1 tsp salt

1 Dissolve the yeast with the sugar in about half the water, or according to the instructions on the packet. Leave to ferment for 10 minutes
2 Sift the flour into a large bowl, make a well in the middle and pour in the yeast mixture, olive

oil and salt. Mix together with a knife and then your hands until it forms a dough

3 Knead the dough for 10 minutes until it is springy and elastic. If it is too soft add a little flour

4 Put the dough in a lightly oiled bowl, cover with a damp tea towel and leave it in a warm, draught-free place for about an hour, until it has doubled in size

5 Tip the dough on to a floured surface, divide into two parts and roll out with a rolling pin

6 Put the dough on a floured baking tray and push into any shape you like.

STAGE 2
CORE INGREDIENT
4–5 vine-ripened tomatoes, chopped

FRUIT/VEGETABLES
3 cloves garlic, chopped (optional)
2 red peppers, chopped
1 red onion, finely sliced

FROM THE CUPBOARD
4 T olive oil
4 T tomato paste
2 T water or stock

HERBS AND SPICES
1 tsp salt

1 Heat the oil, sauté the onion for 2 to 3 minutes then add the garlic, tomato paste and peppers and continue to sauté for another 2 to 3 mins

2 Add the tomatoes, salt and stock and continue to cook for about 15 minutes, stirring occasionally and squashing the tomato against the sides of the pan.

STAGE 3
FRUIT/VEGETABLES
12 marinated artichoke hearts
12 olives, chopped

FROM THE CUPBOARD
4–6 T pesto (page 118)
1 T olive oil

HERBS AND SPICES
2 T fresh basil

1 Spread the pesto over the top of the pizza base

2 Cover with the tomato mixture

3 Add artichoke hearts and chopped olives and drizzle over a little extra olive oil and bake in a preheated 220°C oven for about 15 to 20 minutes until the exposed dough is golden brown

4 Sprinkle with fresh basil leaves.

PREPARATION TIME:
15 minutes, plus 60 minutes
rising time/COOKING TIME:
35–40 minutes

OTHER PIZZA TOPPINGS
Pesto and tomato sauce with:
● Spinach, and roasted
vegetables
● Leeks and green beans
● Pineapple and corn
● Anchovies and capers
● Caramelised onions and olives

TORTILLAS (3)
CORE INGREDIENT
Tortillas

FRUIT/VEGETABLES
shredded lettuce
4 tomatoes, sliced
2 avocados, peeled and sliced
1 T lemon juice

FROM THE CUPBOARD
4 T hummus

HERBS AND SPICES
chilli sauce

1 Warm the tortillas in the oven
2 Spread hummus (page 107)
down the centre of the tortilla
3 Top with lettuce, tomatoes
and avocado tossed in lemon
juice
4 Add chilli sauce to taste
5 Roll up tortilla and serve.

PREPARATION TIME:
10 minutes/COOKING TIME:
2–3 minutes

VARIATION:
● *Fill with baked beans.*

**SUGGESTED FAMILY
RECIPES**
● Any pasta dish
● Fried rice
● Bacon, potato, avocado and
tomato stacks
● Kedgeree
● Any stir-fried dish
● Duck in Chinese pancakes
● Chicken and rice

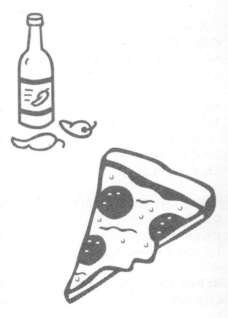

9 Away days

- *Keep focused and determined*
- *Take key ingredients with you*
- *Always be alert for dairy*

Perhaps the most difficult situations for keeping to the Plant Programme arise when you are away from home – eating out or travelling. Here is some advice to help you to cope in such situations. To some extent it is all a matter of confidence. Make up your mind that you are being sensible and rational and do not allow yourself to be teased or persuaded to eat dairy, processed or junk food. **Stick to your guns!**

9.1 HOSPITAL

This is probably the most difficult place to obtain the kind of food that we recommend – especially state-run hospitals in the UK. Nonetheless, hospitals **should** provide vegan meals. We recommend that you order these and keep your own supplies of fresh organic fruit and vegetables to top up with and to ensure that you have lots of healthy vitamins. It is a good idea to take soya 'milk' with you for your cereal. Most hospitals have refrigerators that patients can use, but remember to label all your food items clearly with your name. Also, avoid that awful milky hospital tea and coffee. Ask for cups of hot water and add delicious green, fruit or herbal teas from packets stowed in your locker.

9.2 EATING WITH FAMILY OR FRIENDS

This is usually easy to deal with. If you have cancer, or have had the disease, most people will want to do everything possible to help. It is simply a matter of giving advance notice and a clear explanation of what you will and will not eat. Give examples of meals that you enjoy, that are relatively simple to prepare. Remember that if people are afraid that it is all too difficult, they may stop inviting you out. Try not to fuss or to make an issue of your diet. If the worst comes to the worst and you are confronted by a meal with, for example, dairy-based sauces ask if you can have your meal without the sauce. If it is too late and the meal has been served simply scrape off the sauce discreetly. Or if, for example, you are given a large slab of cheesecake for dessert ask quietly and politely if you could have a piece of fresh fruit instead. You will soon find everyone copes with your needs without question and some will even start to follow a similar regime!

9.3 RESTAURANT EATING

Most large cities have vegetarian restaurants that also specialise in vegan food. Some have a mission statement committing them to using organically produced ingredients. Many other restaurants have a vegetarian option, although you need to check carefully, ideally with the chef, that this does not contain dairy.

French restaurants can be the most difficult. The ones we have tried simply do not understand the concept of a non-dairy diet, let alone vegan meals. In the case of European restaurants in general, the best way of ensuring a meal free of dairy is to say you are allergic (it may not be that far from the truth!). That raises the spectre of lawyers and lawsuits and ensures they will do their best. However, even well-meaning chefs can still make mistakes. For example, we have been given vegetable soup that tasted of that inimitable 'cow taste'. Upon enquiring, we discovered that it was made using commercially available whey, which the chef did not know was dairy produce (**had he forgotten about Little Miss Muffet?**).

Oriental (Chinese, Korean, Japanese, Thai) restaurants are usually the best sources of non-dairy meals, although many Indian restaurants use dairy, including yoghurt, in curries and other dishes. Unfortunately many Chinese (and some Indian) restaurants now buy food prepared in a factory. In the worst cases, they buy whole meals in plastic bags that are reheated, or (worse!) microwaved before serving. We call this '**fossil food**'. It is the antithesis of real oriental food that aims to use the freshest possible ingredients. If a restaurant has a very large number of dishes on the menu and you cannot smell cooking smells, or hear cooking noises coming from the kitchen, be suspicious. It is often small unpretentious restaurants in the Chinese sector of cities where real Chinese meals can be found. Seek out and be prepared to pay for good food made with fresh ingredients, rather than eat factory food in flashy surroundings.

In general, Japanese restaurants are particularly good, because often the meal is prepared in front of you. Most of the Korean or Thai restaurants in which we have eaten use fresh ingredients. Whether eating out in a Western or Asian restaurant, it is usually a good idea to choose from the 'specialities of the house', or the daily blackboard specials. These are most likely to be made on the spot from fresh ingredients, and least likely to contain '**fossil food**'.

Wherever you choose, it is always a good idea to telephone or visit the restaurant ahead, in order to avoid having to make an issue about your meal, when you simply want to eat good food and enjoy yourself with friends or family. We find that our favourite restaurants are always prepared to help us select dishes or make modifications to meals so that we can enjoy eating, while keeping to our programme.

9.4 FAST FOOD AND SNACKS

In Chapter 6, we suggested that you should make and take snacks and light meals with you when you are on the move. This is not always possible, so here is some advice to help you make the healthiest choices when you are out and about.

Pizzerias are usually good for a light hot meal, especially if you are with children and teenagers. Most will prepare any pizza from their range **without cheese** and they usually have good tasty salads.

Fish and chip shops are fine for an occasional treat, provided the food is fried in fresh oil and cooked in breadcrumbs. If the fish is cooked in batter simply remove it before eating the fish. If you have a local 'chippy' ask if they will make batter with soya milk for you – they will often do this for a regular customer.

Lebanese and other Middle Eastern cafes are a good source of dairy-free food that is fresh and tasty.

NEVER eat burgers, sausages or other foods that could have been prepared from mechanically recovered meat, that is sucked off the carcasses of dead dairy cows or chickens (yuck!).

Cold snacks can be found fairly easily, but most sandwich breads and rolls usually contain dairy produce in some guise. Check the ingredients list carefully and remember that many spreads, margarines and commercial mayonnaise can contain hidden dairy. Baguettes frequently have no butter or butter substitutes spread on them and are therefore a better bet. We like sandwich bars where you can have baguettes or sandwiches made up with the ingredients of your choice in front of you. Ask for them to be wrapped in paper, **NOT** plastic or clingwrap.

Salads can be relatively easy to find. They are available pre-packed in many large stores and supermarkets, or they can be made up individually in some delicatessens and the delicatessen sections of some supermarkets, and paid for according to weight.

Delicatessens are a good source of healthy tasty ingredients to make your own snacks. They often sell artichoke hearts, sun-dried tomatoes, or fat green olives in olive oil, hummus, mushroom pâtés, and delicious breads. Delis are especially useful in the United States, where it can be particularly difficult to find healthy snacks and light meals.

Japanese-style lunch boxes usually provide good dairy-free snacks. A particularly good vegetarian sushi lunch box is available from outlets of a large chain that sells ready to eat food.

Buy drinks in glass, metal or cardboard containers, **NEVER** in plastic bottles. Drink from glasses or pottery cups or mugs. For hot drinks, order herbal or green tea. If it is not available ask for a cup of hot water and add your own herbal tea sachet.

9.5 ON THE MOVE

Some preparation is needed if you are to keep to your programme while travelling. A minimum survival kit includes enough brewer's yeast, kelp and red clover tablets to cover for the entire time away, and a small pot of dried soya 'milk' (normally sold in cans for babies and infants). Take herbal and green tea bags and enough fresh fruit to see you through until you can find a local supply.

It is difficult to buy healthy food when travelling by train or coach. We suggest you carry your own, or stock up at a good shop

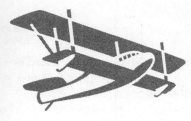

before boarding.

When flying ensure you have pre-ordered dairy-free meals, and check that the travel agent uses the correct code. VGML is the code for vegan food with no dairy; AVML is the code for Asian vegetarian food, which is also non-dairy and is often spicy; while ORML is the code for oriental food which is non-dairy, but is likely to contain some meat. Vegetarian meals with the code VLML are likely to contain considerable quantities of dairy produce, which is used to replace meat. A light meal consisting entirely of fruit has the code FPML.

Before you travel it might be worth trying to find a hotel that serves organic and vegan food using websites, such as HotelsTravel.com. Also look up key words in a dictionary and jot them down in the language of the country you will be visiting. In France, for example 'soya' is 'soja'. Having a small number of ready-translated words to hand will be of great help during your visit. Ask your hotel where to buy the items you need, using the written version if necessary. There will often be a supermarket, shop or market near your hotels where you can buy supplies, including beer, coincidentally avoiding the hotel's expensive minibar.

Travelling in China (but not necessarily Hong Kong), Japan, Thailand and Korea used to mean you could relax, knowing all the food fitted the Programme. However, Western food is increasingly popular, so choose carefully and do not be afraid to ask questions.

When you arrive at your destination, locate the nearest fruit and vegetable stall or shop and buy fresh supplies daily. In many countries fruit and vegetables must be put in boiling water before eating. Briefly immerse all of the items using the hotel sink as soon as you return from shopping, but do be careful not to scald yourself.

Research the local cuisine and check out those dishes that you will be able to eat without problem or fuss. Tell everyone you are terribly allergic to dairy produce and if all else fails, scrape off the yoghurt, butter, cream, etc. Be inventive – for example, use fruit juices to moisten your cereal rather than milk.

10 Food as Medicine*

People can suffer from a range of side effects as a result of the various types of cancer treatment. Being in hospital, where there is a concentration of sick people, sometimes in old buildings that are difficult to clean, can also lead to infections – especially in those whose immunity may have been impaired by chemotherapy.

Here is a list of some of the most effective methods of dealing with health problems caused by breast cancer treatments, or other treatments, without resorting to pills and potions, many of which contain dairy products. Even Tamoxifen tablets are usually in a lactose (milk sugar) base.

Even people who are not suffering from cancer can benefit from changing to the Programme described in this book. Making the simple modifications to the basic Plant Programme described below can treat the common conditions listed, even though they are unrelated to cancer.

Just one thing before you begin this section – we have assumed you have cut out all dairy produce from your diet, otherwise we would have to repeat – **'CUT OUT DAIRY'** for every ailment! As a general tip, bathe or shower at least once each day, and put on clean underwear afterwards. It is good for morale and helps keep down infection.

SYMPTOM:
ACHING JOINTS AND LIMBS AND ARTHRITIC SYMPTOMS

CAUSE: Often a side effect of chemotherapy.

DIET
Reduce the acidity and increase the alkalinity of your system:
● *Replace citrus fruits and berries* *with melon, apples, pears, apricots, mangoes or bananas*
● *Replace tomatoes and beetroot with red peppers*
● *Increase the amount of celery, celery seeds and parsley in your diet*
● *Avoid malt vinegar and use small quantities of cider vinegar instead*
● *Drink real ales rather than wines or spirits and camomile or*

ALWAYS discuss your symptoms with your physician, especially if they are severe or persistent.

*peppermint tea rather than fruit
teas, coffee or black tea*
● *Eat some oily fish because it is
anti-inflammatory (ensure you eat
only wild fish from unpolluted
sources).*

TIPS
● *Avoid pH-balanced gels, soaps
or shampoos. Use simple soap and
Epsom salts in your bathwater*
● *Chronic symptoms unrelated to
cancer may benefit from
glucosamine sulphate and
chondroitin sulphate supplements
(it is possible to buy products
suitable for vegans)*
● *Learn to move and lift correctly
and to adopt the correct posture*
● *Ensure you are not overweight*
● *Acupuncture can be helpful and
massaging with rosemary oil is
said to be soothing.*

*SYMPTOMS CAUSED BY
CHEMOTHERAPY
SHOULD RESPOND TO
THESE SIMPLE CHANGES
IN DIET AND LIFESTYLE
IN A WEEK OR SO.*

SYMPTOM: **ALLERGIES
INCLUDING ASTHMA,
SINUSITIS AND RHINITIS
AND ECZEMA**

CAUSE: Sometimes made worse
by cancer treatment

DIET
● *Garlic, onion, horseradish and
citrus fruit help reduce mucus*
● *Oily fish can help but ensure it
is wild.*

*THANK GOODNESS YOU
NO LONGER HAVE DAIRY
PRODUCE, WHICH IS ONE
OF THE COMMONEST
UNDERLYING CAUSES OF
ALLERGIES.*

SYMPTOM: **ANAEMIA
REFLECTED BY DIZZINESS,
PALLOR, FATIGUE AND/OR
LOSS OF APPETITE**

CAUSE: Sometimes a side effect
of chemotherapy

DIET
● *Ensure you have your brewer's
yeast*
● *Add lots of iron-rich herbs such
as dandelion, nettle, parsley and
watercress (which are also rich in
calcium) to salads and soups*
● *Eat lots of grapes especially red
and black ones.*

SYMPTOM: **APPETITE LOSS**

CAUSE: Often a side effect of chemotherapy

DIET
If this is just for a day or so after chemotherapy it is probably your liver and kidneys needing a rest to recover. If the loss of appetite persists it could be because of low cobalt or zinc levels so:
● Ensure you take your brewer's yeast
● Eat sesame and pumpkin seeds and tahini
● Eat an occasional egg, the yolks are a good source of minerals.

FOLLOW THE ADVICE FOR SICKNESS AND DIARRHOEA AND THEN GRADUALLY INTRODUCE THE FOODS YOU FIND MOST APPEALING. BE GUIDED BY YOUR SENSE OF SMELL. IT IS A VERY GOOD GUIDE.

TIPS
● Make sure food is presented attractively
● If you are in hospital and the food is unappetising try to arrange for friends or family to bring in your meals.

SYMPTOM: **CHEST INFECTION WITH COUGHING AND DIFFICULTY IN BREATHING**

CAUSE: Viral or bacterial infection

DIET
● Increase intake of garlic, onions and chives.

TIPS
● Inhale menthol, oil or essence of tea tree, eucalyptus or thyme available from most good pharmacists. Add a few crystals or drops of the oil or essence to very hot water, put a towel over your head and inhale deeply.

SYMPTOM: **COLD SORE**

CAUSE: Herpes virus activated by below par immune system

DIET
● Eat garlic, onions and chives
● Rosemary and ginger are also said to improve the immune system.

TIPS
● Rub with fresh garlic at the first tingle and do it again frequently. This will cause the cold sore to

disappear more quickly
● *Wear lipstick or an UV barrier cream to keep away sunlight which helps to stimulate the virus.*

SYMPTOM: **CONSTIPATION, HAEMORRHOIDS AND VARICOSE VEINS**

CAUSE: Can occur as a result of anxiety and as a side effect of some anti-nausea and some antidepressant tablets. Iron tablets also cause constipation. The pressure of a full, congested bowel on blood vessels draining the lower abdomen and legs causes haemorrhoids and, in some cases, varicose veins.

DIET
● *Organic linseed is particularly helpful*
● *Figs and pears are some of the best fruits for this condition*
● *Asparagus is a natural laxative especially if you eat the stems as well as the tips.*

IT'S GOOD YOU NO LONGER EAT CHEESE – REMEMBER ITS OLD NICKNAME WAS BUNG!

TIPS
● *Exercise is helpful.*

SYMPTOM: **CONVALESCENCE IN GENERAL**

DIET
Extra Miso soup. This is used by the Japanese as a cure-all in the same way that Jewish people use chicken soup. The recipe for this delicious soup is on page 52.

SYMPTOM: **CUTS AND BRUISES**

CAUSE: Normal accident but take extra care to avoid infection

TIPS
● *Tea tree oil is a powerful but gentle antiseptic that relieves pain and stimulates healing*
● *Infusions made with a few Marigold flowers from the garden dabbed on the wound help bites, stings, aches, boils and cuts to heal.*

SYMPTOM: **CYSTITIS**

CAUSE: Can be caused by an infection because of a below par immune system or by irritation of the bladder as a result of excretion of chemotherapeutic drugs (or radiotherapy in the case of prostate cancer)

DIET
● *Whatever the cause, drink lots of filtered boiled water.*
If your urine is thick, bubbly or especially smelly it is likely to be an infection. In that case:
● *Drink barley or cranberry juice to encourage frequent bladder emptying and fight infection. Cranberry juice is thought to prevent bacteria sticking to the walls of the urinary tract so they are easier to flush out*
● *Asparagus and celery are also natural diuretics.*
If there is no indication of infection:
● *Reduce the acidity in your diet by following the advice for aching bones and joints and arthritis above*
● *Do not take cranberry or barley water, which are acid. Instead mix some Soya baby formula in warm water to alkalise and calm down the irritation in your bladder*
● *Cut out black tea, coffee, alcohol, sugar and spices.*

TIPS
● *Wear cotton pants and wash at high temperature*
● *Women should wear stockings and suspender belts rather than tights*

● *After bowel movements wipe from anus towards base of spine to avoid carrying bacteria near to the opening of the bladder. Follow up by washing thoroughly in a bidet whenever possible*
● *Follow the advice for bathing described under aching joints and limbs.*

SYMPTOM: **DEPRESSION AND ANXIETY INCLUDING IRRITABILITY, SLEEPLESS-NESS, POOR CONCENTRAT-ION AND FATIGUE**

CAUSE: Many people with cancer suffer from depression and anxiety so do not be embarrassed to ask for help

DIET
● *Reduce alcohol and eliminate caffeine*
● *To ensure you have adequate B vitamins take brewer's yeast*
● *Improve your zinc levels by eating pumpkin seeds and sesame seeds or tahini*
● *Have lots of miso soup (page 52)*
● *A diet high in starchy foods such as bread, pasta and especially brown rice and low in (especially refined white) sugar steadies blood sugar levels which can cause mood swings*

● *Banana, nuts and turkey contain an amino acid that stimulates production of serotonin a brain chemical that improves mood*
● *Camomile tea soothes anxiety while peppermint is said to enliven the brain improving clarity of thought*
● *Dark chocolate is especially good because it triggers release of endorphins the body's 'feel good' chemicals, but buy only organic dairy-free brands or make your own chocolate soya 'milk' (page 224–5).*

TIPS
● *Force yourself to exercise regularly to increase the level of 'feel good' chemicals in the brain*
● *Enjoy a long period of natural light each day*
● *Spend time with friends and family members whose presence you find comforting but try not to wear individuals down too much*
● *Try to sort out any underlying problems in your life and ask for professional help in developing coping methods for those that cannot be resolved*
● *Herbal remedies include Borage, Lavender, St John's Wort and Vervain, but these are not recommended during chemotherapy and it is always wise to consult a professional*

herbalist
● *A few drops of lavender oil added to your bath water or dropped on your pillow is said to improve mood.*

SYMPTOM: **FLUID RETENTION WITH SWOLLEN BREASTS AND BLOATED FEELING**

CAUSE: Caused by hormone treatment or before periods

DIET
● *Asparagus, celery, cranberry juices are especially helpful*
● *Ensure you take your brewer's yeast and kelp tablets.*

SYMPTOM: **FUNGAL INFECTIONS BETWEEN THE TOES OR IN THE ARMPITS**

CAUSE: Fungi thrive in warm, moist, dark conditions

DIET
● *Increase your intake of garlic, onions and chives.*

TIPS
● *Keep affected area dry with high-quality talc and expose to the*

sun and air as much as possible
● Try dabbing with cotton wool
soaked in tea tree oil (never use
the cotton wool twice)
● Wear cotton clothing and wash
it at a high temperature.

SYMPTOM: **HEADACHE**

CAUSE: Often caused by stress
and anxiety. Sometimes the
result of dehydration following
sickness or simply being in a
hot dry hospital.

DIET
● Rehydrate and relax the blood
vessels around the brain by
drinking lots of diluted fresh
vegetable and fruit juices.

SYMPTOM: **HEART PROBLEMS**

CAUSE: Can be exacerbated
by chemotherapy

DIET
● Oily fish is good
● Again garlic is helpful. It
improves circulation, reduces
clotting and helps lower blood
pressure
● Globe artichokes are also good

for the heart. They also increase
bile production and help break
down fat.

THE PLANT PROGRAMME DIET IS HEART HEALTHY.

TIPS
● Meditation to reduce stress
lowers cholesterol.

SYMPTOM: **HOT FLUSHES AND OTHER MENOPAUSAL SYMPTOMS**

CAUSE: Can be caused by
induction of the menopause
by surgery or radiotherapy or
as a side effect of hormone
treatments for cancer

DIET
● Ensure your diet contains
enough good sources of
phytoestrogens such as soya,
beans, nuts, whole grains –
especially linseed or flax and
sprouting seeds such as alfalfa
and berries
● Try clover teas
● Sage teas help menopausal
symptoms but do not drink them
if there is any chance you are
pregnant
● Celery, cranberry and
asparagus are natural diuretics

that help to deal with fluid retention including before periods.

SYMPTOM: **ITCHING SKIN**

CAUSE: Side effect of some drugs

TIPS
● *Tepid baths with starch or a little baking soda can be soothing*
● *Calamine lotion is also soothing and good for the skin*
● *Work with your physician to identify the drug causing the symptoms and ask to try a good alternative.*

SYMPTOM: **MOUTH ULCERS**

DIET
● *Brewer's yeast again and other good sources of B vitamins such as whole grains and potatoes.*

SYMPTOM: **NAIL INFECTIONS**

DIET
● *Increase intake of garlic, onions and chives.*

TIPS
● *Soak frequently in warm, salty water.*

SYMPTOM: **OSTEOPOROSIS**
(A skeletal disorder of progressive bone mass loss and demineralisation causing increased risk of fracture)

CAUSE: We have included this condition because many women have been persuaded they need to consume dairy produce to obtain sufficient calcium. This is NOT the case.

DIET
● *In general keep to a diet with a high ratio of food of vegetable origin to that of animal origin*
● *Eat lots of dark green vegetables such as kale, broccoli, spinach and watercress*
● *Eat plenty of fruit, especially berries, figs, kiwifruit and oranges*
● *Eat plenty of nuts, seeds and tofu*
● *Reduce caffeine and alcohol intake*
● *If you must have alcohol keep to real ales*
● *Oily fish is helpful.*

TIPS
● *Ensure you have regular exercise*
● *Sunshine and daylight helps vitamin D levels important for strong and healthy bones.*

SYMPTOM: **SICKNESS AND DIARRHOEA**

CAUSE: Caused by chemotherapy or gastro-intestinal infection

DIET
● *As soon as you are able to keep drinks down sip filtered, boiled water*
● *If the symptoms persist ask the pharmacist for powders to re-balance your electrolytes*
● *Take occasional sips of warm water to which you have added the contents of a lactobacillus capsule (do not eat the gel capsule). This will repopulate the gut with good bacteria after chemotherapy and compete with any bad bacteria that are causing sickness and diarrhoea*
● *Eat bread and other dry cereals when you feel able to do so to soak up the toxins produced by infection*
● *Rice, especially brown rice, is effective against diarrhoea and it helps keep blood sugar levels stable*

● *Thyme, fennel and ginger can help clear infections but use only the fresh herb or spice, not extracts or other medicinal products.*
● *Camomile and peppermint teas are soothing*
● *Drink lots of diluted fresh vegetable and fruit juices as soon as you are able*
● *Olive oil is said to stimulate cleansing of the gallbladder*
● *Pineapple, papaya and onions and garlic help to breakdown fats.*

TIPS
● *Always wash hands thoroughly*
● *If it is an infection wash towels, bed linen and underwear in a hot wash.*

SYMPTOM: **SKIN SORENESS/BURNING**

CAUSE: Occurs at the later stages of radiotherapy

DIET
● *Ensure good zinc status by munching lots of pumpkin and sesame seeds*
● *Spread tahini on bread and potatoes*
● *Eat lots of fruit and vegetables*
● *Olive oil in your diet will also help healing.*

TIPS
● *Some people find applying aloe vera cream helpful, but make sure it contains no irritating preservatives*
● *Keep washing of the infected area to a minimum to leave any natural oils in your skin. Use tepid water with no soap from a low-power shower*
● *Wear soft, clean white cotton next to the affected area.*

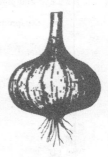

SYMPTOM: **SORE THROAT**

CAUSE: Caused by a virus or bacterial infection

DIET
● *Increase intake of garlic, onions and chives.*

TIPS
● *Gargle frequently with warm, salty water.*

SYMPTOM: **WARTS**

CAUSE: Caused by a virus

TIPS
● *Rub with garlic or lemon juice.*

INDEX OF RECIPES